Dx/Rx: Colorectal Cancer

Kyle Holen, MD

University of Wisconsin Comprehensive Cancer Center
Madison, WI

Ki Young Chung, MD

Memorial Sloan-Kettering Cancer Center
New York, NY

Manish A. Shah, MD
Series Editor

Memorial Sloan-Kettering Cancer Center
New York, NY

JONES AND BARTLETT PUBLISHERS

Sudbury, Massachusetts

BOSTON TORONTO LONDON SINGAPORE

World Headquarters
Jones and Bartlett Publishers
40 Tall Pine Drive
Sudbury, MA 01776
978-443-5000
info@jbpub.com
www.jbpub.com

Jones and Bartlett Publishers Canada
6339 Ormindale Way
Mississauga, Ontario L5V 1J2
Canada

Jones and Bartlett Publishers International
Barb House, Barb Mews
London W6 7PA
United Kingdom

Jones and Bartlett's books and products are available through most bookstores and online booksellers. To contact Jones and Bartlett Publishers directly, call 800-832-0034, fax 978-443-8000, or visit our website, www.jbpub.com.

Substantial discounts on bulk quantities of Jones and Bartlett's publications are available to corporations, professional associations, and other qualified organizations. For details and specific discount information, contact the special sales department at Jones and Bartlett via the above contact information or send an email to specialsales@jbpub.com.

Production Credits
Executive Publisher: Christopher Davis
Associate Editor: Kathy Richardson
Production Director: Amy Rose
Production Assistant: Leah Corrigan
Associate Marketing Manager: Rebecca Wasley
V.P. of Manufacturing and Inventory Control: Therese Connell
Composition: ATLIS Graphics
Cover Design: Anne Spencer
Printing and Binding: Malloy, Inc.
Cover Printing: Malloy, Inc.

Library of Congress Cataloging-in-Publication Data
Holen, Kyle.
Dx/Rx. Colorectal cancer / Kyle Holen and Ki Young Chung.
p. ; cm. — (Dx/Rx oncology series)
Includes bibliographical references.
ISBN-13: 978-0-7637-4744-2 (alk. paper) 1. Colon (Anatomy)—Cancer—Handbooks, manuals, etc. 2. Colon (Anatomy)—Cancer—Treatment—Handbooks, manuals, etc. 3. Rectum—Cancer—Handbooks, manuals, etc. I. Chung, Ki Young. II. Title. III. Title: Colorectal cancer. IV. Series: Jones and Bartlett Publishers Dx/Rx oncology series.
[DNLM: 1. Colorectal Neoplasms—therapy. WI 529 H729d 2008]
RC280.C6H65 2008
616.99'4347—dc22

2007022430

The authors, editor, and publisher have made every effort to provide accurate information. However, they are not responsible for errors, omissions, or for any outcomes related to the use of the contents of this book and take no responsibility for the use of the products and procedures described. Treatments and side effects described in this book may not be applicable to all people; likewise, some people may require a dose or experience a side effect that is not described herein. Drugs and medical devices are discussed that may have limited availability controlled by the Food and Drug Administration (FDA) for use only in a research study or clinical trial. Research, clinical practice, and government regulations often change the accepted standard in this field. When consideration is being given to use of any drug in the clinical setting, the health care provider or reader is responsible for determining FDA status of the drug, reading the package insert, and reviewing prescribing information for the most up-to-date recommendations on dose, precautions, and contraindications, and determining the appropriate usage for the product. This is especially important in the case of drugs that are new or seldom used.

6048

Printed in the United States of America
11 10 09 08 07 10 9 8 7 6 5 4 3 2 1

Dedication

Dedicated to my colleagues and patients at the University of Wisconsin Comprehensive Cancer Center, as well as my endlessly supportive family.

K.H.

This book is also dedicated to all the patients at Memorial Sloan-Kettering Cancer Center and my family (Rachel, Buddy & Pearl).

K.Y.C.

Contents

Editor's Preface

Welcome to the Dx/Rx Oncology Series. This recently developed series forms a set of handbooks that focus on the practical management of common malignancies. The current handbook, *Dx/Rx: Colorectal Cancer,* is an important handbook in the collection given the recent explosion of new drugs available for the management of colorectal malignancies. This handbook provides a comprehensive, yet succinct overview of the diagnosis and management of colon and rectal cancer. Together, these diseases are amongst the most common malignancies in the world. Our improving understanding of biology, and the resultant recent development of targeted agents that affect angiogenesis or inhibit epidermal growth factor receptor signaling have significantly improved patient outcomes and have affected our management of the disease in recent years. In a time span of about 15 years, we have made significant progress, improving median survival by 100% from about 12 months to about 24 months. The future of the management of this disease is as bright. This handbook provides a succinct, yet comprehensive foundation for you as the management of this disease evolves over the next several years. The bulleted format unique to this new series allows for quick access to vital and practical management issues for your patients' treatment. Drs. Holen and Chung have put together a handbook that will serve as an essential resource to you and your practice. I know you will find this and several of the books in this series to be invaluable for your everyday use and patient care.

Manish A. Shah, MD

Preface

There are approximately 110,000 new cases of colon cancer and another 30,000 cases of rectal cancer diagnosed in the United States each year, accounting for approximately 20% of all cancers diagnosed. With a mortality of over 50,000, colon and rectal cancers are the second leading cause of death from cancer among men and women. Fortunately, there have been dramatic improvements in colorectal cancer treatments over the last few years, resulting in significant improvements in both the length and quality of life for patients. In fact, there have been more new chemotherapies approved for colon and rectal cancer in the last 5 years than for any other cancer.

Here, Dr. Chung and I will not only present the latest advances in the field but provide a review of the most important revelations in the field since 1954, the year Dr. Heidleberger first published his report on 5-fluorouracil.

Kyle Holen, MD

CHAPTER 1

Epidemiology

Incidence and Mortality

- The American Cancer Society estimates that approximately 147,000 people will be diagnosed with colon and rectal cancer in the United States in 2004. This is the fourth highest cancer incidence, after prostate, breast, and lung cancers.[1]
- Of these 147,000 people, 40,570 will be diagnosed with rectal cancers.
- Approximately 57,000 people will die from colon and rectal cancers in 2004. This is the second leading reason for cancer deaths, after lung cancer.
- The incidence and mortality from colon and rectal cancers is about equal in men and women.
- The mean age at diagnosis is between 60 and 65, with over 90% of all cases diagnosed in people over the age of 50.
- Countries in Asia, Africa, and Latin America have a lower incidence of colorectal cancer than those in North America and Western Europe. The rate of the lowest incidence population group (Gambia) at 0.7 per 100,000 is dramatically different from the rate of the highest incidence population group (Japanese men in Hawaii) at 37.2 per 100,000.

Etiology and Risk Factors

Diet

- There has been a long debate as to the role of fat and fiber in one's diet and the risk of colorectal cancer. Around the world, countries in Asia, Africa, and Latin America that have a low-fat, high-fiber diet have a much lower incidence of colon cancer as compared to countries in North America and Europe that have a high-fat, low-fiber diet. Those who adhere to a vegetarian diet have also been documented to have a lower incidence of colon cancer. Interestingly, immigrants from Japan to the United States have a colon cancer rate 2.5 times that of their native Japan counterparts. The mechanisms of high fiber aiding in preventing colon cancer are thought to be secondary to the decreased amount of time the stool is in the colon and the general diluting and absorption of possible carcinogens. A high-fat diet results in changes in the gut microflora and increases the concentration of fecal bile acids.

- Prospective trials, however, have yet to show any relation between diet and colon cancer risk. Four large studies from Japan, Israel, and the United States have failed to show a relationship between either meat or fat intake and colonic malignancy. Controversy continues regarding fiber and its role in preventing colorectal cancers. Several studies have shown inverse relationships between fiber intake and colon cancer incidence.
- The Nurses' Health Study was initiated in 1976 when 121,700 female registered nurses who were 30 to 55 years of age and residing in the United States completed a mailed questionnaire on known or suspected risk factors for cancer. They were then followed every other year with questionnaires regarding changes in dietary intake or new diagnoses of cancer. From this cohort, there were no associations between the intake of dietary fiber and the risk of colorectal cancer.[2] Studies in men also have failed to show an association between fiber intake and colon cancer.[3]
- The Women's Health Initiative (WHI) was a prospectively designed study where women ages 50 to 79 years were randomly assigned to a dietary modification group (40%, $n = 19{,}541$) or a comparison group, who were not asked to make dietary modifications (60%, $n = 29{,}294$).[4] The women in the dietary modification group were asked to consume a reduced amount of fat (20% of energy) and an increased amount of vegetables and fruits (five or more servings a day) and grains (six or more servings a day). Over the 8.1 years of follow-up, there were 201 cases of invasive colorectal cancer (0.13% per year) in the intervention group and 279 (0.12%) in the comparison

group. This difference was not statistically significant. The WHI low-fat eating pattern intervention did not reduce the risk of invasive colorectal cancers. There was no evidence of reduced risk for any category of colorectal cancer outcome associated with the intervention. Evidence from this study strongly suggests that lowering dietary fat intake and increasing fruit, vegetable, and fiber intake in mid to late life cannot be expected to reduce the risk of colorectal cancer in this length of time.

Genetic Factors

- There are clear genetic susceptibilities associated with colon cancer. However, even without detectable genetic abnormalities, children and siblings of those diagnosed with colon cancer remain at increased risk. The general concept of all inherited colon cancers follows the multistep model created by Fearon and Vogelstein.[5] The model outlines the multiple genetic mutations that need to occur when normal colonic mucosa progresses to adenomas, carcinomas, and eventually metastatic disease. In such a model, those who inherit mutations would need fewer acquired mutations in order to progress to colon cancer. See Figure 1-1.

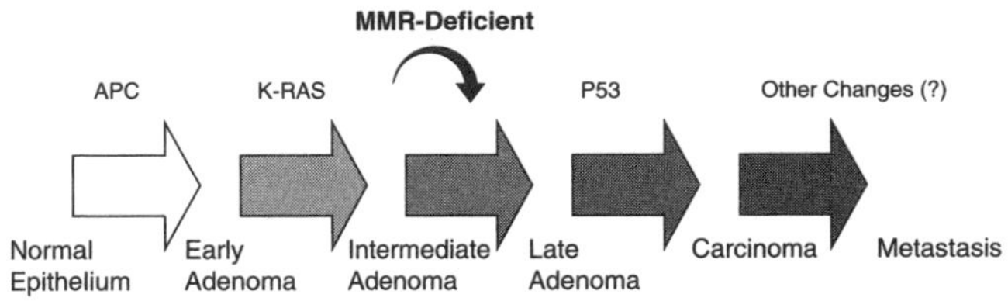

Figure 1-1: Genetic Changes Associated with Colorectal Tumorigenesis. A cellular transition occurs from normal colon epithelium to adenoma to invasive cancer. APC mutations are believed to initiate tumor progression, with the development of other mutations as indicated in the diagram. Individuals with FAP inherit APC mutations and thus have already begun this pathway earlier than the general population. HNPCC tumors go through a similar process and MMR mutations are believed to accelerate this process. K-ras is an oncogene that requires only one mutation for activation, whereas the other specific genes in the diagram are tumor suppressor genes that are recessive at a cellular level (require two mutations before loss of tumor suppression occurs). Adapted from *Lessons from Hereditary Colorectal Cancer*, 97:159–170, Oct 1996.

Table 1-1: Modified Bethesda Guidelines for MSI Testing: Tumors from Any of the Following Should Be Tested for MSI (or by Immunohistochemistry) and then Positive Patients Should Continue for MMR Testing

■ CRC < age 50 years
■ Synchronous or metachronous colorectal or other HNPCC-associated tumors regardless of age
■ CRC with MSI-positive morphology < age 60 years
■ CRC with one or more first-degree relatives with CRC or other
■ HNPCC-related tumor, with one of the cancers < age 50 years
■ CRC with two or more first- or second-degree relatives with CRC or other HNPCC-related tumor (regardless of age), including cancers (endometrial, stomach, ovarian, cervical, esophageal, leukemia, thyroid, bladder, ureter and renal pelvis, biliary tract, small bowel, breast, pancreas, liver, larynx, bronchus, lung, and brain [glioblastoma], sebaceous gland adenomas, and keratoacanthomas)

Abbreviations: MMR, mismatch repair; CRC, colorectal cancer; HNPCC, hereditary nonpolyposis colon cancer; MSI, microsatellite instability.

- Familial adenomatous polyposis (FAP), a germline mutation in the APC gene on chromosome 5q, has been shown to cause extensive, on the order of hundreds to thousands, of polyps throughout the gastrointestinal tract. It is autosomal dominant with a very high penetrance. About 30% of people without a family history have FAP, suggesting that there is a fairly high rate of spontaneous mutations. The gene frequency is on the order of 1 in 5,000 to 1 in 25,000. People with this mutation are recommended to undergo prophylactic complete colectomy to avoid a near certain diagnosis of colon cancer in their future, commonly before the age of 50.
- Hereditary nonpolyposis colorectal cancer (HNPCC) is associated with defects in mismatch repair enzymes leading to microsatellite instability in the tumor. HNPCC is characterized by early-onset carcinomas of the large

bowel and endometrium, with more modest increases in risk of cancers at other sites. The Amsterdam Criteria or Bethesda Guidelines have historically been used to assess a patient's risk for HNPCC with limited success. See Tables 1-1 and 1-2. Recently, Lipton et al. have suggested using an improved, quantitative algorithm to assess for risk of microsatellite instability, called the Amsterdam plus model.[6] In most models, you estimate the risk of a hereditary syndrome. With a higher risk, you then assess the tumor for microsatellite instability. If microsatellite instability exists, then you proceed to the more expensive and complicated testing of a germline mutation of hMSH2, hMLH1, hPMS1, hPMS2, or other genes associated with microsatellite instability.

- Those with HNPCC have predominantly right-sided lesions, and therefore may not have as high a risk of rectal cancers.
- First-degree family members of those diagnosed with colorectal cancer, even without a history of HNPCC or FAP, still have a five times greater risk of colon cancer than those without a family history. Therefore, a discussion of

Table 1-2: Amsterdam Criteria II: All of the Following Must Apply for a Putative Diagnosis of HNPCC to Be Made in a Family

■ There are at least three relatives with an HNPCC-associated cancer (large bowel, endometrium, small bowel, ureter, or renal pelvis, though not including stomach, ovary, brain, bladder, or skin)
■ One affected person is a first-degree relative of the other two
■ At least two successive generations are affected
■ At least one person was diagnosed before the age of 50 years
■ Familial adenomatous polyposis has been excluded
■ Tumors have been verified by pathologic examination

Abbreviation: HNPCC, hereditary nonpolyposis colon cancer.

Table 1-3: The Relationship Between Possible Risk Factors and Colonic Neoplasm*

Risk	Odds Ratio (95% CI)
Age	
50–54	1.00
>60	3.83 (2.39 – 6.14)
Sex	
M	1.00
F	0.65 (0.33–1.29)
Race	
W	1.00
B	0.84 (0.53–1.34)
Family History	
No relatives with colon cancer	1.00
≥ 2 relatives with colon cancer	3.00 (1.23–7.30)
NSAID Use	
Never	1.00
Daily or more	0.65 (0.48–0.89)
Physical Activity†	
24–28	1.00
29–36	0.86 (0.63–1.16)
> 36	0.67 (0.49–0.93)
Smoking	
Never	1.00
Current	2.12 (1.49–3.01)
Alcohol	
Never	1.00
Current	1.53 (1.07–2.17)

*From Lieberman, et al. *JAMA* 2003, 290: 2959–2967.

†Physical activity scores were tabulated by scoring the number of hours of activity in categories of very light, light, moderate, and heavy to achieve a 24 hour score. The higher the score, the higher the level of activity.

adequate screening for family members is essential for all those diagnosed with colorectal cancer.

Physical Activity

- A marginal association between physical activity and colonic neoplasms was noted in a 2003 study of over 3,196 patients who underwent a colonoscopy.[7] In the study, 1,441 patients without polyps were compared to the 329 patients who had a neoplastic lesion. The age-adjusted odds ratio for those who said they had no exercise vs. those who had vigorous activity was 0.67, with confidence intervals of 0.49 to 0.93. See Table 1-3 for more results regarding this study.

Inflammatory Bowel Disease

- The higher risk of colon cancer for patients with ulcerative colitis and Crohn's disease is well documented. Such patients must have frequent screening, and if a tumor is detected, should strongly consider a full colectomy. Colon cancers as a result of inflammatory bowel disease do not behave differently than routine colon cancers. Risk is associated with length of time with the disease, from 3% risk in the first decade to 30% in the third decade.

Other Risk Factors

- Retrospective analyses have suggested the following possible risk factors: smoking,[7,8] obesity, and exposure to various materials including asbestos and organic solvents.

References

1. American Cancer Society. *Cancer facts and figures 2004.* New York: American Cancer Society; 2004.
2. Fuchs CS, Giovannucci EL, Colditz GA, et al. Dietary fiber and the risk of colorectal cancer and adenoma in women. *N Engl J Med.* 1999;340:169–176.
3. Platz EA, Giovannucci E, Rimm EB, et al. Dietary fiber and distal colorectal adenoma in men. *Cancer Epidemiol Biomarkers Prev.* 1997;6:661–670.

4. Beresford SAA, Johnson KC, Ritenbaugh C, et al., Low-fat dietary pattern and risk of colorectal cancer: The Women's Health Initiative Randomized Controlled Dietary Modification Trial. *JAMA*. 2006;295:643–654.
5. Vogelstein B, Fearon ER, Hamilton SR, et al., Genetic alterations during colorectal-tumor development. *N Engl J Med*. 1988;319(9):525–532.
6. Lipton LR, Johnson F, Cummings C, et al. Refining the Amsterdam Criteria and Bethesda Guidelines: testing algorithms for the prediction of mismatch repair mutation status in the familial cancer clinic. *J Clin Oncol*. 2004; 22:4934–4943.
7. Lieberman DA, Prindiville S, Weiss DG, et al. Risk factors for advanced colonic neoplasia and hyperplastic polyps in asymptomatic individuals. *JAMA*. 2003;290:2959–2967.
8. Chao A, Thum MJ, Jacobs EJ, Henley SJ, Rodriquez C, Calle EE. Cigarette smoking and colorectal cancer mortality in the cancer prevention study II. *J Natl Cancer Inst*. 2000; 92:1888–1896.

CHAPTER 2

Prevention and Screening

Chemoprevention

- Efforts are underway to determine, in a prospective fashion, whether nonsteroidal anti-inflammatory drugs (NSAIDs) can reduce the risk of colorectal cancer. COX-2 inhibitors have been shown to reduce the number of polyps for those with familial adenomatous polyposis (FAP). Because of this, the Adenomatous Polyp Prevention on Vioxx (APPROVe) study was designed to determine rofecoxib's effect on benign sporadic colonic adenomas, and ultimately on the incidence of colorectal cancer. Late in 2004, rofecoxib was withdrawn from the market by Merck, following the premature cessation, by the data and safety monitoring board, of the APPROVe trial due to a significant increase (by a factor of 3.9) in the incidence of serious thromboembolic adverse events in the group receiving 25 mg of rofecoxib per day, as compared with the placebo group.[1]
- The Nurses' Health Study has shown that those with regular aspirin use had a lower risk of colorectal cancer.[2] As mentioned in the VA study[3] in Chapter 1, Table 1-3, patients who used a nonsteroidal anti-inflammatory drug once or more daily had a slightly lower risk of neoplastic polyps, with an odds ratio of 0.63 (95% CI 0.48–0.98).
- Aspirin use has also been evaluated in a higher risk population, specifically those with a diagnosis of stage III colon cancer who were enrolled in a study evaluating adjuvant therapy with fluorouracil and leucovorin with and without irinotecan. In this study, a medical history was obtained both prior to enrollment and 6 months after adjuvant therapy was completed on the 846 patients enrolled. Those who were taking aspirin on both surveys were considered consistent aspirin users. After adjusting

for age, gender, performance status, T-stage, N-stage, bowel perforation, bowel obstruction, baseline serum carcinoembryonic antigen (CEA), tumor differentiation, adjuvant treatment arm, and other NSAID use, consistent aspirin users had a hazard ratio for disease recurrence of 0.45 (95% CI 0.21–0.96). This did not seem to be dependent on the dose of aspirin used; however, the small numbers of patients precluded statistical analysis.[4]

Screening

- See Table 2-1 for a list of recommendations from the American Cancer Society.
- *Digital rectal exam (DRE):* The digital rectal exam is of little value if used alone as a screening method for colon cancer, in that it can only detect tumors 7–8 cm from the anal verge. It is estimated that fewer than 10% of colorectal cancers can be palpated by the examining finger, with all of these being rectal cancers. It is easy to do, however, and can be done as part of the fecal occult blood test (FOBT), a test recommended by many physician organizations.

Table 2-1: Screening Guidelines from the American Cancer Society Facts & Figures 2004

Screening Test	Frequency
FOBT or FIT	Annual
Flexible Sigmoidoscopy	Every 5 years
FOBT or FIT with Sigmoidoscopy	Annual and every 5 years; this combination is recommended over either test alone
Double Contrast Barium Enema	Every 5 years
Colonoscopy	Every 10 years*

*Recommended every 5–10 years if no polyps noted on exam. Courtesy of American Cancer Society.

- *FOBT and fecal immunochemical testing (FIT):* The U.S. Preventive Services Task Force recommends annual FOBT for those over age 50, based on a randomized controlled trial showing decreased mortality from colorectal cancer in those who underwent FOBT screening. The American Cancer Society, the American Gastroenterological Association, and the American College of Obstetricians and Gynecologists have also recommended annual FOBT.

  FIT detects the globin portion of hemoglobin, which does not survive past the upper GI tract and therefore may have fewer false positive results than seen from FOBT. There is not a consensus regarding the routine use of FIT at this time.
- *Sigmoidoscopy:* Sigmoidoscopy also has been shown to reduce mortality from colorectal cancer and is recommended by the U.S. Preventive Health Services Task Force. This screening test, however, is not very sensitive. More than 40% of colon cancers are missed due to the inability to evaluate cancers in the transverse and right colon.
- *Colonoscopy:* The sensitivity of colonoscopy is much higher than the previously mentioned screening tests, and is therefore recommended for those with a prior diagnosis of colon cancer, those with inflammatory bowel disease, those with a strong family history of colon cancers, and those with multiple polyps noted on prior enteroscopies. Prospective studies are ongoing to prove disease-specific mortality impact from colonoscopy. Images of cancer and benign polyps are shown in Figure 2-1. Findings on colonoscopy range from benign sessile or pedunculated polyps to cancerous polyps and large tumors. Obstructing mass lesions require emergent surgery.
- *Barium enema:* A noninvasive way to image the colon. It is limited in that those with positive tests must then undergo colonoscopies.
- *Virtual colonoscopy:* A virtual colonoscopy (also known as colonography) uses computed tomography scans through the colon to assess for polyps or other suspicious lesions. This CT scan requires a complete bowel prep for adequate visualization, similar to the prep required prior to

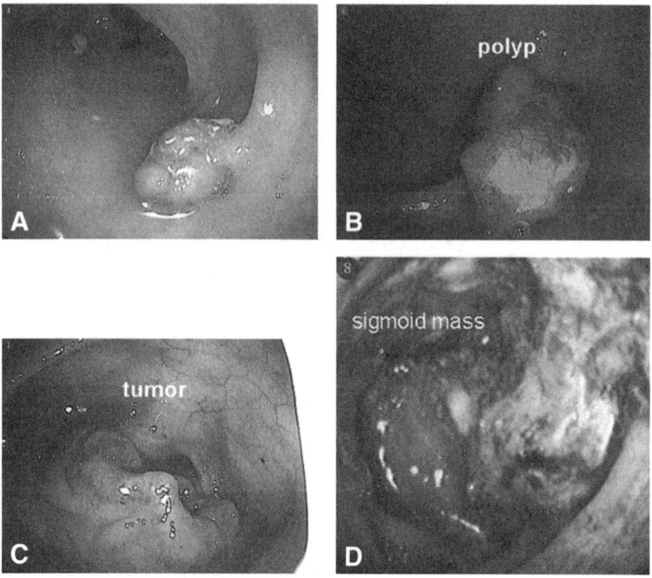

Figure 2-1: Benign polyp, cancerous polyp, and a malignant tumor as viewed by optical colonoscopy. A pedunculated, benign tubulovillous adenoma is shown in (A), while a cancerous polyp with evidence of bleeding and mucosal disruption is shown in (B). The tumor in (C) is a well-differentiated adenocarcinoma, as is the tumor in (D); however, the tumor in (D) has obstructed the lumen of the sigmoid colon and needs emergent surgery.

optical colonoscopy. Pickhardt and colleagues have published the sensitivity (93.8%) and specificity (96.0%) of virtual colonoscopy.[5] This test has yet to show a decrease in disease-specific mortality in a randomized trial; however, the sensitivity and specificity are equivalent to optical colonoscopy. Like the barium enema, this test is limited by the fact that it is a diagnostic tool only. Patients with a positive test must then have a colonoscopy to evaluate polyps or other abnormalities. Advantages to the test include lower risk of bowel perforation and the ability to see abnormalities outside the wall of the colon. Images from a virtual colonoscopy are seen in Figure 2-2.

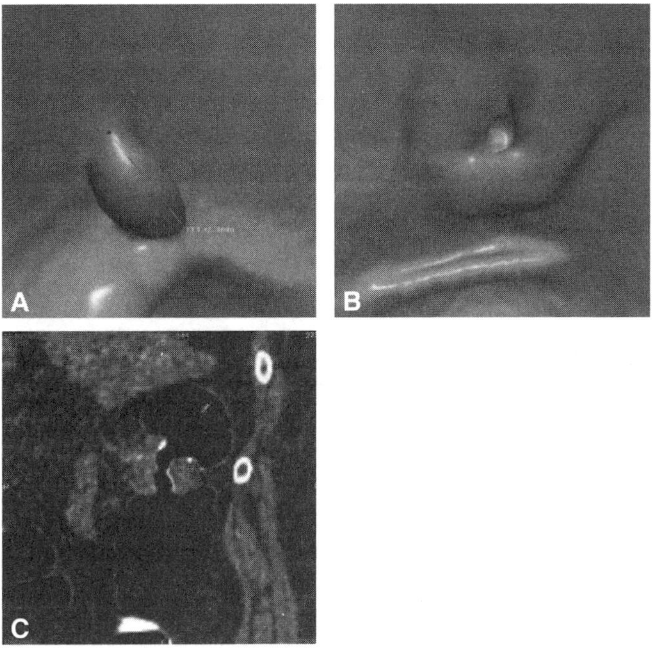

Figure 2-2: Images from virtual colonoscopy (colonography). In (A), the colonography shows a pedunculated polyp, measuring 1.3 cm. A tumor is seen in figure (B), and the coronal image (C) shows the tumor as a classic "apple core" lesion.

References

1. FitzGerald GA. Coxibs and cardiovascular disease. *N Engl J Med.* 2004;351(17):1709–1711.
2. Chan AT, Giovannucci EL, Schernhammer ES, et al. A prospective study of aspirin use and the risk for colorectal adenoma. *Ann Intern Med.* 2004;140(3):157–166.
3. Lieberman DA, Prindiville S, Weiss DG, Willett W; VA Cooperative Study Group 380. Risk factors for advanced colonic neoplasia and hyperplastic polyps in asymptomatic individuals. *JAMA.* 2003;290(22):2959–2967.
4. Fuchs C, Meyerhardt JA, Heseltine DL, et al. Influence of regular aspirin use on survival for patients with stage III colon cancer: findings from Intergroup trial CALGB 89803.

Abstract #3530, American Society of Clinical Oncology Annual Meeting, June 2005.

5. Pickhardt PJ, Choi JR, Hwang I, et al. Computed tomographic virtual colonoscopy to screen for colorectal neoplasia in asymptomatic adults. *N Engl J Med.* 2003;349:2191–2200.

CHAPTER 3

Pathology, Staging, and Prognosis

Pathology

- The overwhelming majority of colon and rectal cancers are adenocarcinomas. Other pathologic descriptions of colon and rectal cancers include mucinous adenocarcinoma (which has more than 50% extracellular mucin), signet-ring cell carcinoma (more than 50% signet ring cells with intracellular mucin production), or poorly differentiated carcinoma. Histologic images are shown in Figure 3-1.
- Rare pathologies of the colon and rectum include neuroendocrine tumors (high grade extrapulmonary small cell tumors or low grade carcinoid tumors), sarcomas including gastrointestinal stromal tumors (GISTs), malignant melanomas of the colon and rectum, and primary colorectal lymphomas. The prognosis, staging, and treatment for these tumors are quite different than for routine adenocarcinomas of the colon and rectum.
- Also uncommon is an entity described as pseudomyxoma peritonei, a slow-growing adenocarcinoma that spreads mainly through the peritoneum. This tumor generally does not respond to systemic chemotherapy and therefore the routine treatment includes debulking of the tumor by surgical resection. Repeat resections are commonly required.
- Vascular invasion and lymphatic invasion predict a higher risk of recurrence after surgery.
- Histologic grading is used to describe the degree of tumor differentiation. See Table 3-1.
- Metastatic spread includes local invasion of the primary tumor into surrounding structures, "drop" metastases into the peritoneum, lymphatic spread through regional lymph nodes, and hematologic spread through the bloodstream to distant organs. Given that the blood return

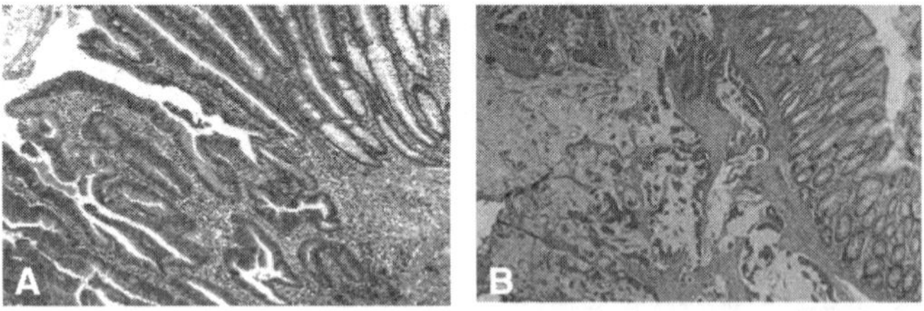

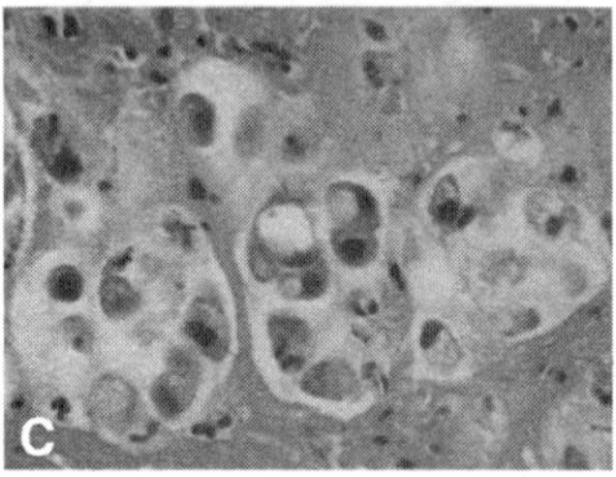

Figure 3-1: Colon cancer histology (A-C).

from the colon first passes the liver, liver metastases are the most common site of distant spread.

TNM Staging and Dukes Staging

- Staging systems are devised to separate patients with high probability of relapse from those with low probabil-

Table 3-1: Histologic Grading of Colon and Rectal Adenocarcinomas

Grade	Description
G1	Well differentiated, a carcinoma with cellular features that closely resemble normal epithelium
G2	Moderately differentiated, cellular features that are in between grades G3 and G1
G3	Poorly differentiated, cells that retain some gland formation or mucous production but only barely resemble normal epithelium
G4	Undifferentiated, cells with no clear recognizable squamous or glandular features

ity, in order to guide further therapy and provide information to the patient regarding prognosis. The most widely used staging systems are the Dukes staging system, modified by Astler-Coller in 1954, and the TNM staging system, proposed by the American Joint Committee on Cancer. The Dukes staging system was most recently modified by the Gastrointestinal Tumor Study Group (GITSG) in order to better prognosticate those with multiple involved lymph nodes, thereby breaking stage C into C1 and C2. See Table 3-2.

- The survival rates correlate well with the staging system. For stage I there is a 90–100% 5-year survival rate, stage II disease has a 60–80% 5-year survival rate, stage III disease has a 42% 5-year survival rate, and stage IV only an 8.5% survival rate. Survival worsens, however, with the associated poor risk factors: histologic grade, lymphatic or blood vessel invasion, elevated carcinoembryonic antigen (CEA), increased number of lymph nodes involved, bowel obstruction or perforation at presentation, African-American race and expression of thymidylate synthase in the tumor.
- In those who present with metastatic disease, an elevated lactate dehydrogenase (LDH) level, a white blood cell (WBC) count greater than 10,000, and a Karnofsky performance status of less than 60 all correlate with a decreased survival rate.
- In a retrospective evaluation of over 3,500 patients with Dukes stage B and C cancers, the extent of the lymph node dissection was correlated with overall survival. In Dukes C patients, the extent of lymph node dissection did not correlate with median overall survival or recurrence rate; however, in patients with Dukes stage B cancer, those with less than seven lymph nodes sampled had a higher rate of recurrent disease and a decrease in survival. This suggests that patients with Dukes B cancer are understaged if fewer than seven lymph nodes are sampled.[1]
- Sentinel lymph node staging has yet to show equivalence to multilevel sectioning in risk stratification for those with early stage tumors.[2]

Table 3-2: TNM/Dukes Staging

T, N, or M Stage		Definition	TNM Stage	Dukes Stage
T				
	Tis	Carcinoma in situ	0	
	T1	Tumor invades submucosa	I	A
	T2	Tumor invades into muscularis propria		B1
	T3	Tumor invades through the muscularis propria	II	B2
	T4	Tumor invades into local structures		B3
N				
	N0	No lymph nodes		
	N1	1–3 lymph nodes involved	IIIA	C1
	N2	4 or more lymph nodes	IIIB	C2
	N3	Lymph nodes identified along a named vascular trunk		
M				
	M0	No distant metastases		
	M1	Distant metastases identified	IV	D

References

1. Prandi M, Lionetto R, Bini A, et al. Prognostic evaluation of stage B colon cancer patients is improved by an adequate lymphadenectomy: results of a secondary analysis of a large scale adjuvant trial. *Ann Surg*. 2002;235(4):458–463.
2. Bertagnolli M, Miedema B, Redston M, et al. Sentinel node staging of resectable colon cancer: results of a multicenter study. *Ann Surg*. 2004, 240(4):624–628.

CHAPTER 4

Early Stage Treatment

Stage I

- Surgery is the only curative treatment required for stage I colorectal cancer.
- Laparoscopic surgical resection has been compared to open colectomy for stage I, II, and III colon cancer. In this study, 872 patients were randomized to receive open colectomy or laparoscopic surgery. Patients with bowel perforation or obstruction, transverse colon lesions, severe medical illness, inflammatory bowel disease, familial adenomatous polyposis (FAP), or metastatic disease were excluded. The patients were well balanced between the two groups in terms of age, sex, location of primary, tumor stage, and tumor grade. Ninety patients originally assigned to laparoscopy were converted during the operation to open colectomy. The group that received laparoscopically assisted colectomy had longer operating room times; however, they had an improved time to recovery and a decrease in narcotic use. More importantly, they had comparable complication and recurrence rates. This type of resection, however, should be advised only in the hands of a surgeon well trained in this procedure and should include a good sampling of regional lymph nodes.[1] See Table 4-1 for results.
- Operative mortality is influenced by the mode of presentation and the nature of the surgical resection. The operative mortality of a resection performed emergently is 20%, compared with only 5% when the procedure is performed electively.[2]
- Total prophylactic colectomy is well established as the necessary treatment for those with longstanding inflammatory bowel disease or FAP. There is ongoing debate regarding the use of prophylactic colectomy for those with

Table 4-1: Recurrence, Disease-free Survival, and Overall Survival Rates After Laparoscopic-assisted Hemicolectomy

Endpoint (4.4 year follow up)	Open Colectomy (n = 428)	Laparoscopically-assisted Colectomy (n = 435)	p value
Recurrence	84 (19.6%)	76 (17.5%)	0.83
Disease-free Survival	311 (72.7%)	317 (72.9%)	0.70
Survival	333 (77.8%)	344 (79.1%)	0.51

Adapted from *NEJM* 2004;350:2050–2059.

hereditary nonpolyposis colorectal cancer (HNPCC) vs. frequent colonoscopic surveillance.

Stage II

- Standard surgery includes a hemicolectomy with lymph node dissection. Please see the previous section on stage I management regarding the use of laparoscopic surgery.
- Adjuvant chemotherapy for patients with stage II colorectal cancer (CRC) remains controversial. Stage II colorectal cancer (T3-4N0M0), as determined by the American Joint Committe on Cancer (AJCC) TNM staging system, accounts for approximately a quarter of patients and has a relatively good prognosis after definitive surgical resection, with a 72%–85% overall survival rate (stage IIA [T3N0M0] 85%; stage IIB [T4NM0], 72%).[3,4] In contrast to the clear survival benefit of adjuvant chemotherapy for node-positive stage III disease, its role in stage II colon cancer remains controversial, because a statistically insignificant 2%–5% improvement in overall survival with adjuvant therapy has been demonstrated from multiple studies. For fit "high risk" stage II patients with clinical obstruction or perforation at presentation in which the 5-year survival rate is 60%–70%, there is little controversy, because these patients are routinely treated

with adjuvant chemotherapy. Other potential high risk factors including high histologic grade, microsatellite instability, and loss of 18q have yet to be validated in prospective trials. Patients with fewer than 12 regional lymph nodes identified in the surgical specimen have a statistically unclear risk of lymph node involvement. These patients may represent stage III disease and should receive adjuvant therapy.

- Multiple randomized trials involving both stage II and stage III colorectal cancer patients have failed to demonstrate a statistically significant survival benefit from 5-fluorouracil (5-FU)–based adjuvant chemotherapy in the subset of patients with stage II cancer. None of these trials, including the North Central Cancer Treatment Group, the International Multicenter Pooled Analysis of Colon Cancer Trials (IMPACT), and the Multicenter International Study of Oxaliplatin/5-FU/LV in the Adjuvant Treatment of Colon Cancer (MOSAIC) trials, was statistically powered to discern small differences in survival.
- Unfortunately, most published adjuvant studies involve both stage II and stage III CRC patients, and hence have not been powered to address small survival differences in the stage II CRC population. Hence, the decision to treat stage II CRC patients relies heavily on subset analyses of adjuvant trials, database studies, and large meta-analyses.

Select Randomized Stage II Colon Cancer Trials

- A subset analysis of 318 stage II patients in U.S. Intergroup 0035 randomized to receive either 5-fluorouracil (5-FU) and levamisole (Ergamisol) or surgery alone demonstrated no difference in 7-year survival rates, 72% for both groups ($p = 0.83$).[5,6]
- The Quick and Simple and Reliable (QUASAR) adjuvant trial from the United Kingdom involving 3,289 resected predominately stage II CRC patients (92%) with "uncertain indications" demonstrated a statistically significant improvement in recurrence rate (22.2% vs. 26.2%; HR 0.78, 95% CI 0.67–0.91) and 5-year survival (80.3% vs. 77.4%; HR 0.83, 95% CI 0.71–0.97) with adjuvant chemotherapy compared to observation.[7] Although a 3%

statistical survival advantage has been demonstrated, this trial was not statistically designed to address the magnitude of benefit of adjuvant chemotherapy specifically for stage II CRC patients.[7]

- The International Multicenter Pooled Analysis of Colon Cancer Trials (IMPACT) investigators attempted to address the role of adjuvant chemotherapy in stage II CRC patients. This pooled analysis from five European trials involving 1,016 stage II colon cancer patients randomized to adjuvant 5-FU/LV versus observation demonstrated a 5-year survival rate of 82% versus 80%, respectively. The hazard ratio for overall survival at 5 years was 0.86 (90% CI 0.68–1.07) and 0.83 (90% CI 0.72–1.07) for disease-free survival, respectively. Hence, this analysis demonstrated a nonstatistically significant 2% survival advantage of adjuvant chemotherapy for stage II CRC patients, suggesting that an observation-only arm remains valid for stage II CRC trials.[8]
- A subset analysis of the MOSAIC Trial involving 899 patients with stage II CRC randomized to adjuvant FOLFOX-4 (oxaliplatin [Eloxatin]/5-FU/LV) or infusional 5-FU/LV (LV5FU2) alone demonstrated no statistically significant advantage of adjuvant FOLFOX-4.[9,10] With a median follow-up of 37.9 months, the stage II patients demonstrated disease-free survival (DFS) rates of 87.0% in the FOLFOX-4 arm and 84.3% in the LV5FU2 arm (HR 0.80, 95% CI 0.56–1.15). Twelve percent (108 of 899) of the stage II patients with high-risk features (T4 lesion, perforation, obstruction, or vascular invasion) also demonstrated no statistical DFS advantage of FOLFOX-4 compared with LV5FU2 (84.9% vs. 79.8%; HR 0.72, 95% CI 0.48–1.08). This study did not have an observation arm, and hence the advantage of chemotherapy over observation for stage II colon cancer patients cannot be determined.[9,10]

Stage II CRC Adjuvant Epidemiologic Evaluations

- The Surveillance, Epidemiology, and End Results (SEER) Medicare Analysis used the Medicare database to identify 3,151 stage II patients with no high risk features. Approximately 27% of these elderly Medicare patients received adjuvant chemotherapy (predominately 5-FU/LV). With an overall survival rate of 78% for chemotherapy patients versus 75% for observed patients, this analysis suggests minimal benefit of adjuvant chemotherapy for stage II CRC patients without high risk features.[11]

Stage II CRC Adjuvant Trial Meta-analyses

- Multiple meta-analyses have attempted to determine the benefit of chemotherapy in stage II CRC patients: The pooled Intergroup Meta-Analysis evaluated 3,302 stage II and III colon cancer patients from seven randomized trials comparing adjuvant 5-FU/LV or 5-FU/Levamisole versus observation. A multivariate analysis adjusted for T-stage, histologic grade, nodal status, and adjuvant 5-FU–based chemotherapy. DFS of 67% versus 55% (HR 0.70; 95% CI 0.63–0.78) and 5-year overall survival rate of 71% versus 64% (HR 0.74; 95% CI 0.66–0.83), respectively, were significantly improved with adjuvant chemotherapy. The advantage of chemotherapy was seen in all subsets, although patients with stage II (node-negative) CRC did not demonstrate a survival advantage (81% vs. 80%, $p = 0.113$).[4]
- The Cancer Care Ontario Practice Guideline Initiative (CCOPGI) Gastrointestinal Cancer Disease Site Group systematically reviewed 37 trials and 11 meta-analyses published after 1987. A separate meta-analysis sanctioned by the American Society of Clinical Oncology (ASCO) was performed on a subset of 12 trials (4,187 patients) with an observation arm and at least one 5-FU–based adjuvant chemotherapy arm for stage II colon cancer patients. The mortality risk ratio for stage II CRC patients did not reach statistical significance (HR 0.87, 95% CI 0.75–1.10, $p = 0.07$).[12]

ASCO and NCCN Guidelines

- The ASCO and National Comprehensive Cancer Network (NCCN) guidelines do not recommend routine administration of 5-FU–based chemotherapy for resected stage II colon cancer patients. Suggestions are made for consideration of adjuvant chemotherapy for medically fit patients with inadequate lymph node sample size (< 12) or high-risk features (T4, perforation, high-grade histology) or consideration of a clinical trial.[13]

Other High-Risk Features of Colon Cancer That Require Further Prospective Evaluation

- Neural and vascular invasion have been reported to be associated with local and distant failure, respectively.[14-16]
- Allelic loss of chromosome 18q in colon tumors has been demonstrated to be a marker of poor prognosis.[17] In a retrospective evaluation of 145 tumor samples for 18q loss, investigators demonstrated a lower 5-year survival rate in 18q-loss patients versus those without 18q loss (54% vs. 93%, respectively). Interestingly, a 52% 5-year survival rate in stage II 18q-loss patients was similar to that for stage III patients without 18q loss.
- Microsatellite stability within colon tumors also appears to predict poor prognosis.[18] In an evaluation of 570 patients from three 5-FU–based adjuvant trials, tumor samples were retrospectively analyzed for microsatellite instability. Among patients who did not receive adjuvant therapy, the 5-year survival rate was significantly better in patients with tumors that exhibited high-frequency microsatellite instability (88.0% vs. 68.4%; $p = 0.004$) than in those patients with tumors exhibiting microsatellite stability or low-frequency instability. Adjuvant chemotherapy improved the overall survival rate of patients with microsatellite-stable tumors or tumors exhibiting low-frequency microsatellite instability ($p = 0.04$), but not those with high-frequency microsatellite instability.
- In contrast, a recent analysis of MSI from archival tissues from four National Surgical Adjuvant Breast and Bowel Project (NSABP) adjuvant CRC chemotherapy trials was conducted. This analysis of NSABP C01-04 trials demonstrated no prognostic correlation between high-degree microsatellite instability and overall survival ($p = 0.67$).[19]

New Trials for Stage II Colon Cancer

- In the NSABP C08 trial, patients with stage II or III disease have been randomly assigned to receive modified FOLFOX-6 for 6 months or modified FOLFOX-6 and bevacizumab for 6 months plus an additional 6 months of bevacizumab. The primary end point is disease-free survival, with secondary end points including safety and overall survival. This study has a 90% power to detect a 25% reduction in risk of relapse after 3 years.
- The Avastin Adjuvant (AVANT) Trial is recruiting 3,450 patients with stage II or III CRC for random assignment to FOLFOX-4 for 6 months or FOLFOX-4 plus bevacizumab 5 mg/kg every 2 weeks for 6 months followed by bevacizumab 7.5 mg/kg every 3 weeks for 6 months, or XELOX (capecitabine/oxaliplatin) plus bevacizumab 7.5 mg/kg every 3 weeks for 6 months followed by bevacizumab at the same dose schedule for 6 months. The primary end point is disease-free survival at 3 years for stage III disease, with the statistical assumption of 80% power to demonstrate a 23% reduction in the hazard ratio. Secondary endpoints include safety, overall survival, pharmacoeconomics, pharmacodynamics, convenience, and satisfaction with treatment.
- The Eastern Cooperative Oncology Group (ECOG) E5202 trial has been designed to evaluate the role of chemotherapy in high-risk stage II CRC patients on the basis of prospective risk stratification for microsatellite stability and 18q status. Patients with microsatellite stability and loss of heterozygosity (LOH) at chromosome 18q are to be randomized to treatment with modified FOLFOX-6 with or without bevacizumab, whereas patients with MSI and no 18q LOH will be assigned to the observation alone arm.
- As we have seen from the irinotecan experience, success in the metastatic setting does not necessarily translate into success in adjuvant therapy. These trials should be actively supported. Until and unless these trials provide positive data, bevacizumab and cetuximab currently have no role in the standard adjuvant treatment of colorectal

cancer, because the relative efficacy and safety of the two agents in this setting remain unknown.

Conclusions

- The decision to use adjuvant chemotherapy to treat low-risk stage II colon cancer patients should be an informed one, comparing an overall survival advantage of 2% to 5% and a 0.5% to 1% risk of mortality with chemotherapy in addition to chemotherapy-related morbidities, such as a 12.4% incidence of grade 3 peripheral neuropathy with oxaliplatin, as well as other morbidities and the anticipated life expectancy of each patient. The available clinical trials and meta-analyses do not clearly settle the issue for or against adjuvant chemotherapy for low-risk stage II colon cancer patients. The current NCCN and ASCO guidelines do not recommend the routine use of adjuvant therapy for low-risk stage II colon cancer patients.
- For perspective, consider the difficulty of similar decisions in other common tumors. For instance, in node-negative breast cancer, which has lower recurrence rates than node-negative colon cancer, patients are routinely given adjuvant chemotherapy based on a net 2% to 7% risk reduction (based on randomized trials of the Early Breast Cancer Trialists' Collaborative Group).[20] This may be mainly because of the larger evidence of benefit and statistical significance of the data, which have convinced the oncologic community of the benefit from adjuvant chemotherapy for node-negative breast cancer.
- We will rely on new adjuvant trials to address many of these clinical questions and to investigate the impact of recently developed therapies to further improve the survival of patients with stage II colon cancer. Thus, at present we must perform a risk-benefit analysis for each individual patient before considering adjuvant chemotherapy for low-risk stage II patients.

References

1. A comparison of laparoscopically assisted and open colectomy for colon cancer. *N Engl J Med.* 2004;350:2050–2059.

2. Scott NA, Jeacock J, Kingston RD. Risk factors in patients presenting as an emergency with colorectal cancer. *Br J Surg.* 1995;82:321–323.
3. Nauta R, Stablein DM, Holyoke ED. Survival of patients with stage B2 colon carcinoma. The Gastrointestinal Tumor Study Group experience. *Arch Surg.* 1989;124:180–182.
4. Gill S, Loprinzi CL, Sargent DJ, et al. Pooled analysis of fluorouracil-based adjuvant therapy for stage II and III colon cancer: who benefits and by how much?. *J Clin Oncol.* 2004;22:1797–1806.
5. Moertel CG, Fleming TR, Macdonald JS, et al. Levamisole and fluorouracil for adjuvant therapy of resected colon carcinoma. *N Engl J Med.* 1990;322:352–358.
6. Moertel CG, Fleming TR, Macdonald JS, et al. Intergroup study of fluorouracil plus levamisole as adjuvant therapy for stage II/Dukes' B2 colon cancer. *J Clin Oncol.* 1995;13: 2936–2943.
7. Gray RG BJ, Hills R. QUASAR: a randomized study of adjuvant chemotherapy vs. observation including 3238 colorectal cancer patients, American Society of Clinical Oncology, 2004.
8. Efficacy of adjuvant fluorouracil and folinic acid in B2 colon cancer. International Multicentre Pooled Analysis of B2 Colon Cancer Trials (IMPACT B2) Investigators. *J Clin Oncol.* 1999;17:1356–1363.
9. Andre T, Boni C, Mounedji-Boudiaf L, et al. Oxaliplatin, fluorouracil, and leucovorin as adjuvant treatment for colon cancer. *N Engl J Med.* 2004;350:2343–2351.
10. Hickish T BC, Navarro M. FOLFOX-4 as adjuvant treatment for Stage II colon cancer: subpopulation data from the MOSAIC trial, American Society of Clinical Oncology, 2004.
11. Schrag D, Rifas-Shiman S, Saltz L, et al. Adjuvant chemotherapy use for Medicare beneficiaries with stage II colon cancer. *J Clin Oncol.* 2002;20:3999–4005.
12. Figueredo A, Charette ML, Maroun J, et al. Adjuvant therapy for stage II colon cancer: a systematic review from the Cancer Care Ontario Program in evidence-based care's gastrointestinal cancer disease site group. *J Clin Oncol.* 2004;22:3395–3407.
13. Benson AB, 3rd, Schrag D, Somerfield MR, et al. American Society of Clinical Oncology recommendations on adjuvant chemotherapy for stage II colon cancer. *J Clin Oncol.* 2004; 22:3408–3419.

14. Compton CC. Pathology report in colon cancer: what is prognostically important? *Dig Dis.* 1999;17:67–79.
15. Horn A, Dahl O, Morild I. Venous and neural invasion as predictors of recurrence in rectal adenocarcinoma. *Dis Colon Rectum.* 1991;34:798–804.
16. Knudsen JB, Nilsson T, Sprechler M, et al. Venous and nerve invasion as prognostic factors in postoperative survival of patients with resectable cancer of the rectum. *Dis Colon Rectum.* 1983;26:613–617.
17. Jen J, Kim H, Piantadosi S, et al. Allelic loss of chromosome 18q and prognosis in colorectal cancer. *N Engl J Med.* 1994;331:213–221.
18. Ribic CM, Sargent DJ, Moore MJ, et al. Tumor microsatellite-instability status as a predictor of benefit from fluorouracil-based adjuvant chemotherapy for colon cancer. *N Engl J Med.* 2003;349:247–257.
19. Kim GP, Colangelo LH, Wieand HS, et al. Prognostic and predictive roles of high-degree microsatellite instability in colon cancer: a National Cancer Institute-National Surgical Adjuvant Breast and Bowel Project Collaborative Study. *J Clin Oncol.* 2007;25:767–772.
20. Clarke M. Meta-analyses of adjuvant therapies for women with early breast cancer: the Early Breast Cancer Trialists' Collaborative Group overview. *Ann Oncol 17 Suppl.* 2006;10:x59–62.

CHAPTER 5

Stage III Treatment and Surveillance

Chemotherapy Rationale

- Patients with stage III CRC have a $\leq$ 50% 5-year survival rate with surgery alone.[1]
- The most important prognostic indicator for survival in locally advanced colon cancer is the stage, as determined by depth of penetration and number of lymph nodes involved, using American Joint Committee on Cancer (AJCC) TNM staging, with subgroups for stages II and III (see Chapter 3, Table 3-2).
- For adequate statistical assessment of lymph node involvement, the current recommendations of the AJCC and the American College of Pathologists are for the examination of at least 12 lymph nodes.[1-3]
- The goal of adjuvant chemotherapy after surgical resection of an early stage colon cancer is to destroy local or metastatic microscopic disease and hence reduce the risk of tumor recurrence and improve survival.
- Over the past 30 years, a series of large prospective, randomized trials have clearly demonstrated the survival impact of adjuvant 5-fluorouracil (5-FU)-based chemotherapy for stage III colorectal cancer patients, with a 30–35% improvement in overall survival rate relative to surgery alone. The role of adjuvant chemotherapy for stage II patients remains unclear, although existing evidence suggests a possible benefit.

Single Agent Fluoropyrimidines

- The clinical benefit of modulated 5-FU regimens in the adjuvant setting of stage III colorectal cancer patients has been established by multiple large prospective randomized trials including the North Central Cancer

Treatment Group (NCCTG) and United States Intergroup 0035 (INT-0035), which have demonstrated a statistically significant 33% risk reduction of death within 1 year with 5-FU/levamisole versus observation.[4,5]

- Further refinement in the schedule of 5-FU administration, 5-FU modulation, and treatment length were determined by Intergroup study 0089 (INT-0089).[6] This trial demonstrated the equivalent risk reduction in stage III patients treated with 6 months of adjuvant bolus 5-FU/LV (Mayo Clinic schedule of daily bolus 5-FU/LV × 5 days every month or Roswell Park schedule of weekly 5-FU/LV × 6 weeks of every 80-week cycle) compared to 1 year of bolus 5-FU/levamisole, with no further added benefit of levamisole to an LV-containing regimen.
- In 1990, the National Institutes of Health (NIH) released a consensus statement recommending that all patients with stage III colon cancer receive adjuvant therapy.[7]
- An oral fluoropyrimidine, capecitabine (Xeloda), which has demonstrated activity and Food and Drug Administration (FDA) approval in the metastatic setting, was formally evaluated in the adjuvant setting in a large prospective randomized trial of 1,987 patients with stage III CRC compared to the Mayo Clinic schedule of bolus 5-FU/LV.[8] This study was statistically powered to demonstrate non-inferiority of capecitabine to the bolus schedule of 5-FU/LV with disease-free survival (DFS) as the primary endpoint. With nearly 4 years of mean follow-up, non-inferiority was demonstrated. In fact, a trend towards improvement in 3-year DFS (HR 0.87; 95% CI 0.75–1.00) and overall survival (HR 0.84; 95% CI 0.69–1.01) was seen. This study suggests that an oral fluoropyrimidine can be substituted for intravenous 5-FU regimens, but does not address the role of combination regimens in the adjuvant setting.

Advanced 5-FU–Based Combination Chemotherapy Regimens

- The FDA-approved chemotherapy agents oxaliplatin and irinotecan have demonstrated synergistic activity with

5-FU and have become the standard of practice in the first and second line treatment of metastatic colorectal cancer patients, based on multiple prospective randomized clinical trials. With these advances in the treatment of metastatic colorectal cancer, it was logical to address the role of these combinations in the adjuvant setting.

Oxaliplatin-Based Adjuvant Therapy

- To determine the benefit of the addition of oxaliplatin to 5-FU/LV for patients with stage II/III colorectal cancer, a large randomized phase III trial (Multicenter International Study of Oxaliplatin/5-FU-LV in the Adjuvant Treatment of Colon Cancer [MOSAIC]) was undertaken involving 2,246 patients.[9] The infusional LV5FU2 regimen was compared to the same regimen plus the addition of oxaliplatin (FOLFOX-4), with a primary endpoint of DFS. Approximately 40% of patients had stage II cancer, 60% with stage III. The overall 3-year DFS for the FOLFOX-4 arm was 78.2% compared with 72.9% for LV5FU2, hence with a 23% risk reduction with FOLFOX-4. In the subset evaluation of stage III patients, the 3-year DFS was 72.2% with FOLFOX-4 versus 65.3% with LV5FU2, with a corresponding 24% risk reduction. The 3-year DFS for stage II patients receiving FOLFOX-4 was 87% compared with 84.3% for LV5FU2, with a net nonstatistically significant 2.7% risk reduction. Toxicities were notable for a 12% incidence of grade 3 sensory neuropathy, which remained at grade 3 in 1% of the patients at the 1-year follow-up.
- The National Surgical Adjuvant Breast and Bowel Project (NSABP) trial C-07 evaluated the addition of oxaliplatin to bolus 5-FU/LV, randomly assigning 2,407 patients with stage II (29%) or stage III colon cancer to three cycles of 5-FU/LV (500 mg/m^2 bolus weekly for 6 of every 8 weeks) with or without oxaliplatin (85 mg/m^2 administered on weeks 1, 3, and 5 of every 8-week cycle). In a preliminary report with a median 34-month follow-up, 3-year DFS for the oxaliplatin/bolus 5-FU/LV arm was 77% versus 72% for bolus 5-FU/LV, with a corresponding 21% risk reduction (HR 0.79). However,

toxicity was prominent in both groups. Hospitalization for diarrhea or dehydration was required in 56 patients receiving oxaliplatin and 34 of the control group, and there were 15 and 14 deaths, respectively, (approximately 1%) during treatment in the oxaliplatin and control groups.[10]

- Based upon the early results of the MOSAIC trial, oxaliplatin was FDA approved, in combination with infusional 5-FU/LV, for the adjuvant treatment of completely resected stage III colon cancer in the United States.

Irinotecan-Based Adjuvant Therapy

- In contrast to oxaliplatin/5-FU/LV trials in the adjuvant setting, which have demonstrated a significant impact in DFS, changing standard practice, trials involving irinotecan in the adjuvant setting have been far less encouraging.
- The Cancer and Leukemia Group B (CALGB) C89803 Intergroup randomized phase III adjuvant trial evaluated the clinical benefit of the weekly irinotecan/5-FU/LV bolus schedule (IFL) versus the bolus Roswell Park 5-FU/LV schedule in patients with stage III colorectal cancer.[11] The addition of irinotecan to bolus 5-FU/LV demonstrated no clinical benefit compared with 5-FU/LV alone in stage III patients. There were no statistically significant differences in DFS and overall survival (OS) between the two arms. A statistically significant higher early death rate was reported for patients randomized to the IFL arm; the 60-day mortality rate was 2.2% in the IFL arm and 0.8% in the Roswell Park 5-FU/LV arm. Significant increases in grade 3/4 neutropenia and febrile neutropenia were identified in IFL arm patients compared with the Roswell Park 5-FU/LV arm (43% vs. 5%, $p < 0.00001$; 4% vs. 1%, $p = 0.08$, respectively). The authors of this study concluded that IFL has no role in the treatment of stage III colon cancer.
- The negative results of the IFL adjuvant study are surprising, and are difficult to explain in the setting of irinotecan's activity and survival advantage in the metastatic setting.

- One hypothesis at the time that the study was first presented was that perhaps the bolus 5-FU schedule was a significant part of the problem, and that the infusional 5-FU regimens might show some benefit in the adjuvant setting.
- The Action to Control Cardiovascular Risk in Diabetes (ACCORD) II trial randomly assigned 400 patients with high-risk stage III disease (four or more nodes positive or obstructed/perforated colon cancers) to biweekly infusional 5-FU/LV with or without irinotecan.[12] In an initial report with median follow-up of 36 months, event-free survival was not significantly different between the arms, but trended towards inferiority of the irinotecan-containing arm. The interpretation of these results is slightly hampered by significant imbalances in important prognostic factors between the arms; there were significantly more patients in the irinotecan group with T3 or T4 primaries, more than 15 positive nodes, vascular invasion, and perineural involvement. However, even in models adjusting for these imbalances, the irinotecan-containing arm remains nonsignificantly inferior.
- It is noteworthy that in a subset analysis of the MOSAIC trial involving FOLFOX, a similar group of high-risk stage III patients (four or more positive nodes) achieved the most benefit from the addition of oxaliplatin, suggesting that this high-risk group would offer the greatest chance for irinotecan to show a favorable result, yet the ACCORD II irinotecan trial is clearly negative.
- The largest trial to evaluate irinotecan in the adjuvant setting is the multicenter Pan-European Trials in Adjuvant Colon Cancer (PETACC)-III trial, which compared infusional 5-FU/LV (biweekly infusion schedule) with and without irinotecan (180 mg/m^2 day 1 every 14 days) in 3,278 patients (2,333 with stage III) with resected colon cancer.[13] In an initial report with a median 32-month follow-up, there was no significant difference in the prespecified primary endpoint of the trial, which was 3-year DFS in the stage III patients (3-year DFS 63% vs. 60%, HR 0.89, $p = 0.107$). A retrospective evaluation of

stage III patients demonstrated a higher percentage of T4 patients in the irinotecan arm compared with the infusional 5-FU/LV alone arm ($n = 180$ vs. 130 patients, 17% vs. 13%). It should be noted, however, that T-stage was not included as a potential prognostic variable for modeling in the protocol; thus its inclusion in the modeling is a post hoc analysis. In this risk-adjusted statistical analysis of the stage III data involving T- and N-stage stratification, a significant DFS (HR 0.85, CI 0.74–0.98, $p = 0.021$) and relapse-free survival rate (HR 0.82, CI 0.71–0.95, $p = 0.009$) was identified. Nonetheless, this trial failed to meet its statistically designed endpoint of improvement of DFS.

- Based upon these three large randomized adjuvant trials, irinotecan-containing chemotherapy appears to be clinically ineffective and should not be considered in routine practice in the adjuvant setting. This is in marked contradistinction to oxaliplatin, which, on the basis of the trials discussed above, should be regarded as appropriate for standard use in the adjuvant treatment of colorectal cancer.

DFS is an Appropriate Endpoint for Adjuvant Studies

- The gold standard for the evaluation of the clinical efficacy for adjuvant therapy trials is the 5-year OS. However, the FDA approved the FOLFOX-4 regimen in the adjuvant setting for stage III CRC based on the improved 3-year DFS. A landmark analysis of 20,898 patients pooled from 18 prospective randomized phase III colorectal cancer adjuvant clinical trials attempted to address the correlation of 3-year DFS to 5-year OS.[14] With an 8-year follow-up, this analysis reported 80% of all recurrence occurring within the first 3 years, and only 5% and 3% of patients recurring in years 4 and 5, respectively. Among the patients disease-free at 3 years, 95% were alive at 5 years, whereas only 9% of patients who demonstrated recurrence in 3 years remained alive at 5 years. The correlation between 3-year DFS and 5-year OS was 0.89 across all trials. Based on this analysis, the Oncology Drug Advisory

Committee (ODAC) to the FDA recommended 3-year DFS as an appropriate endpoint for the evaluation of adjuvant colorectal cancer trials.

Molecular Markers

- At present, we do not have any validated markers to assist in the selection of chemotherapy in the adjuvant setting. Numerous large scale efforts are ongoing, however, to identify molecular characteristics of tumors that will identify them as more or less sensitive to individual chemotherapy agents. Pharmacogenomic studies are attempting to identify those patients who may be at higher risk from toxicity from specific agents. These studies may identify subgroups for whom one therapy or another will be more effective, safer, or both. However, this remains an investigational approach at this time.

Summary

- The administration of a 5-FU/LV–based adjuvant chemotherapy regimen for 6 months demonstrates a clear clinical benefit in patients with stage III CRC. All stage III patients should be offered adjuvant chemotherapy irrespective of age, unless significant comorbity precludes safe administration.
- The FOLFOX regimen is the current standard of practice for stage III CRC patients based on the significant 7% improvement in 4-year DFS.
- The oral fluoropyrimidine capecitabine also appears to be reasonable in patients considered for single agent adjuvant therapy, whereas the role of capecitabine plus oxaliplatin in combination in the adjuvant setting remains to be determined.

Integration of Targeted Agents into Clinical Trials

- Therapeutic options for metastatic colorectal cancers have rapidly expanded with the incorporation of molecularly targeted agents, more than doubling the survival rate of patients.

- Bevacizumab (Avastin), a humanized monoclonal antibody against vascular endothelial growth factor (VEGF) ligand, has demonstrated improvement in objective response rate (RR), progression-free survival (PFS), and overall survival (OS) in combination with cytotoxic chemotherapy, compared to chemotherapy alone. Based on large prospective, randomized clinical trials, bevacizumab is FDA approved in the first and second line setting of metastatic colorectal cancer.
- Cetuximab, a chimeric monoclonal antibody directed against the epidermal growth factor receptor (EGFR), has demonstrated activity as a single agent and in combination with chemotherapy, especially in irinotecan refractory patients, leading to FDA approval in February 2004. Recent preliminary clinical trial data appear to demonstrate significant activity of cetuximab in the first-line setting.
- These targeted agents and others are currently in investigation in combination with chemotherapy in several adjuvant trials.

New Adjuvant Trials for Stage III Colon Cancer

- In the NSABP C08 trial, patients with stage II or III disease are randomly assigned to receive modified FOLFOX-6 for 6 months or modified FOLFOX-6 and bevacizumab for 6 months plus an additional 6 months of bevacizumab. The primary end point is disease-free survival, with secondary end points including safety and overall survival. This study has a 90% power to detect a 25% reduction in risk of relapse after 3 years.
- The Avastin Adjuvant (AVANT) Trial is recruiting 3,450 patients with stage II or III CRC for random assignment to FOLFOX-4 for 6 months or FOLFOX-4 plus bevacizumab 5 mg/kg every 2 weeks for 6 months followed by bevacizumab 7.5 mg/kg every 3 weeks for 6 months, or XELOX (capecitabine/oxaliplatin) plus bevacizumab 7.5 mg/kg every 3 weeks for 6 months followed by bevacizumab at the same dose schedule for 6 months. The primary end point is disease-free survival at 3 years for stage III disease, with the statistical assumption of 80% power to demonstrate a 23% reduction in the hazard ra-

tio. Secondary endpoints include safety, overall survival, pharmacoeconomics, pharmacodynamics, convenience, and satisfaction with treatment.

- The Eastern Cooperative Oncology Group (ECOG) E5202 trial has been designed to evaluate the role of chemotherapy in high-risk stage II CRC patients on the basis of prospective risk stratification for microsatellite stability and 18q status. Patients with microsatellite stability and loss of heterozygosity (LOH) at chromosome 18q are to be randomized to treatment with modified FOLFOX-6 with or without bevacizumab, whereas patients with MSI and no 18q LOH will be assigned to the observation alone arm.
- The North Central Cancer Treatment Group (NCCTG) N0147 trial is randomizing stage III CRC patients to modified FOLFOX-6 with or without weekly cetuximab for 6 months, with disease-free survival as the primary end point. Similarly, the PETACC 8 trial is comparing FOLFOX-4 with or without weekly cetuximab for 6 months, with DFS as the primary end point. These trials and a myriad of other adjuvant trials will continue to address the role of chemotherapy for patients with stage II and III CRC.
- As we have seen from the irinotecan experience, success in the metastatic setting does not necessarily translate into success in adjuvant therapy. These trials should be actively supported. Until and unless these trials provide positive data, bevacizumab and cetuximab currently have no role in the standard adjuvant treatment of colorectal cancer, because the relative efficacy and safety of the two agents in this setting remain unknown.
- Chapter 7 contains a lengthy discussion regarding the chemotherapies mentioned in this chapter. Please refer to Chapter 7 for clarification if necessary.

Surveillance

- The American Society of Clinical Oncology panel on colorectal cancer surveillance recommended a carcinoembryonic antigen (CEA) test every 2–3 months for 2 years

Table 5-1: ASCO Surveillance Guidelines

Test	Comments
History and Physical	Although there is no clear evidence to suggest improved survival and detection of recurrent disease, it is recommended to be done every 3–6 months
Carcinoembryonic antigen (CEA)	It is recommended to test CEA every 2–3 months for 2 years post diagnosis
Fecal occult blood tests	There are insufficient data to recommend routine FOBTs
Computed tomography (CT)	There are insufficient data to recommend routine CT scans
Colonoscopy	All patients should have a complete colonoscopy perioperatively to document a cancer and polyp-free colon. It is then recommended to have a colonoscopy every 3–5 years to detect new cancers and polyps

Courtesy of ASCO.

postdiagnosis, a history and physical exam every 3–6 months, and a colonoscopy every 3–5 years. See Table 5-1.

- A recent study found that patients with frequent radiographic studies (CT) and biochemical evaluations (CEA levels) as part of a surveillance program were more often candidates for metastatic resection than those who did not have radiographic studies (CT), although a survival benefit was demonstrated in this study.[15]

References

1. Greene F PD, Fleming I. The AJCC Staging Handbook (ed sixth). New York, Springer, 2002.
2. Compton CC. Pathology report in colon cancer: what is prognostically important?. *Dig Dis.* 1999;17:67–79.
3. Compton CC. Updated protocol for the examination of specimens from patients with carcinomas of the colon and rectum, excluding carcinoid tumors, lymphomas, sarcomas,

and tumors of the vermiform appendix: a basis for checklists. Cancer Committee. *Arch Pathol Lab Med.* 2000;124: 1016–1025.
4. Moertel CG, Fleming TR, Macdonald JS, et al. Levamisole and fluorouracil for adjuvant therapy of resected colon carcinoma. *N Engl J Med.* 1990;322:352–358.
5. Moertel CG, Fleming TR, Macdonald JS, et al. Intergroup study of fluorouracil plus levamisole as adjuvant therapy for stage II/Dukes' B2 colon cancer. *J Clin Oncol.* 1995;13: 2936–2943.
6. Le Voyer TE, Sigurdson ER, Hanlon AL, et al. Colon cancer survival is associated with increasing number of lymph nodes analyzed: a secondary survey of intergroup trial INT-0089. *J Clin Oncol.* 2003;21:2912–2919.
7. NIH consensus conference. Adjuvant therapy for patients with colon and rectal cancer. *JAMA.* 1990;264:1444–1450.
8. Twelves C, Wong A, Nowacki MP, et al. Capecitabine as adjuvant treatment for stage III colon cancer. *N Engl J Med.* 2005;352:2696–2704.
9. Andre T, Boni C, Mounedji-Boudiaf L, et al. Oxaliplatin, fluorouracil, and leucovorin as adjuvant treatment for colon cancer. *N Engl J Med.* 2004;350:2343–2351.
10. Wolmark N WH, Kuebler JP, et al. A phase III trial comparing FULV to FULV + oxaliplatin in stage II or III carcinoma of the colon: Results of NSABP Protocol C-07, American Society of Clinical Oncology, 2005.
11. Saltz LB ND, Hollis D, et al. Irinotecan plus fluorouracil/leucovorin (IFL) versus fluorouracil/leucovorin alone (FL) in stage III colon cancer (intergroup trial CALGB C89803). American Society of Clinical Oncology, 2004.
12. Ychou M RJ, Douillard J, et al. A phase III randomized trial of LV5FU2+CPT-11 vs. LV5FU2 alone in adjuvant high risk colon cancer (FNCLCC Accord02/FFCD9802), American Society of Clinical Oncology, 2005.
13. Van Cutsem E LR, Hossfeld D. Randomized phase III trial comparing infused irinotecan/5-fluorouracil (5-FU)/folinic acid (IF) versus 5-FU/FA (F) in stage III colon cancer patients (pts). (PETACC 3), American Society of Clinical Oncology, 2005.
14. Sargent DJ, Wieand HS, Haller DG, et al. Disease-free survival versus overall survival as a primary end point for adjuvant colon cancer studies: individual patient data from 20,898 patients on 18 randomized trials. *J Clin Oncol.* 2005;23:8664–8670.

15. Chau I, Allen MJ, Cunningham D, et al. The value of routine serum carcino-embryonic antigen measurement and computed tomography in the surveillance of patients after adjuvant chemotherapy for colorectal cancer. *J Clin Oncol.* 2004;22:1420–1429.

CHAPTER 6

Oligometastatic Disease: Surgical and Regional Approach

Surgery

- Long-term survival can be obtained by resection of isolated liver and lung metastases, with a 25–30% 5-year survival rate reported by institutional series.
- Cryoablation and radiofrequency ablation of finite metastatic liver lesions can result in local control in select patients. These procedures are usually adjuncts to surgical resection. Prospective randomized trials and long-term follow-up are needed to determine the impact of these procedures on local control and overall survival.
- A clinical risk score (CRS) predicting the outcome of patients after hepatic resection of metastatic disease has been developed by Yuman Fong et al.[1] See Table 6-1.
- The use of PET scanning prior to surgical resection of liver metastases has been commonly used to detect occult metastases. A study by Schussler-Fiorenza et al. has shown that PET scans were able to detect extrahepatic disease not seen by CT scanning in 14% of the patients studied who had a CRS of 1 or greater.[2] For those with a CRS of 0, there were no patients with extrahepatic disease determined by PET scans, whereas 57% had false positive readings. The authors, therefore, recommended PET scans only for those patients with a CRS ≥ 1 or suspicious extrahepatic lesions on CT scan.
- Recent debate has focused on the timing of resection of liver lesions in patients with synchronous metastases (patients diagnosed with liver metastases during the identification of the primary tumor). The utilization of chemotherapy prior to resection (neoadjuvant chemotherapy) potentially provides a response surrogate reflecting the biology of the disease, which if effective as demonstrated by a radiologic response, may represent

Table 6-1: Fong Clinical Risk Score

Score One Point for Each Risk Factor: node-positive primary, disease free interval < 12 mos, > 1 tumor, size > 5 cm, CEA > 200 ng/ml

Score	5YS %	Median Survival (mos)
0	60	74
1	44	51
2	40	47
3	20	33
4	25	20
5	14	22

Dr. Fong, et al. *Annals of Surgery,* 1999;230:309. Used with permission from Lippincott, Williams, and Wilkins.

elimination of local and extralocal microscopic disease below the threshold of radiologic studies, and hence potential for definitive curative resection. Additionally, neoadjuvant chemotherapy allows for a tailored approach to additional adjuvant therapy provided after the surgery. However, converse arguments include a possible increase in operative morbidity/mortality with neoadjuvant chemotherapy as well as the possibility of missing a therapeutic window of possible resection of chemotherapy refractory disease.

- Unfortunately, no large prospective randomized trial has been performed or will likely ever be practically performed to address the optimal approach, based on the relative infrequency of oligometastatic disease and the heterogeneity of presentations and chemotherapy choices in these patients.

Hepatic Artery Infusion

- There remains conflicting evidence regarding the use of hepatic artery infusion (HAI) chemotherapy after surgical resection to reduce the risk of recurrent disease. The premise of HAI-based therapy is based on the dual blood supply of the liver, with metastatic tumors deriving more than 85% of their blood supply from the hepatic artery, whereas the normal liver parenchyma derives much of its blood supply from the portal vessels.

Adjuvant Therapy After Resection of Hepatic Metastases

- Patients who undergo resection of liver metastases from colorectal carcinoma have a significant survival advantage. However, the majority of patients will relapse frequently within the liver. Attempts at risk reduction with adjuvant therapy are warranted, modeling the significant risk reduction of adjuvant chemotherapy for stage III colorectal adenocarcinoma.
- Adjuvant 5-FU (fluorouracil) systemic chemotherapy alone has not been shown to have a significant survival benefit in liver-metastases resected patients in several clinical trials.
- A German cooperative multicenter trial randomized 226 patients to resection alone or resection plus HAI 5-FU/LV provided as a 5-day continuous infusion every 28 days.[3] This study was terminated early because a survival benefit of HAI 5-FU/LV (leukovorin) was extremely unlikely based on interim data. The interpretation of this trial is difficult because only 74% of patients were actually treated in the HAI arm and only 30% of patients actually completed the 6 months of therapy. No differences in Time to Tumor Progression (TTP) or overall survival were seen in an intention-to-treat analysis, although a trend towards improved disease-free survival was seen. See Table 6-2.
- An American Intergroup trial randomized 109 patients to resection alone or resection followed by four cycles of HAI floxuridine (FUDR) plus systemic 5-FU, and an additional four cycles of systemic 5-FU alone.[4] No statistically significant difference in overall survival was seen in this trial. However, of the 109 randomized, only 80 actually entered the trial. When these 80 patients were analyzed, there was a statistically significant increase in

Table 6-2: Randomized Trials of Adjuvant HAI Chemotherapy After Complete Resection of Liver Metastases

Study	German 1998		MSKCC 1999		Intergroup 2002	
Arms	HAI FUDR + IV 5-FU/LV	IV 5-FU/LV	HAI FUDR IV 5-FU/LV	No tx	HAI 5-FU/LV	No tx
N	113	113	74	82	53	56
N (%) receiving Assigned tx	84 (74)	100 (88)	68 (92)	76 (93)	30 (57)	45 (80)
Median TTP (mo)	20	12.6	37.4*	17.2	37**	18**
Median OS (mo)	44.8	39.7	72.2	59.3	63.7	49.7
2-year PFS	NR	NR	57%	42%	46%	25%
2-year HPFS	67% 1.5 year HPFS	63%	90%*	60%	67%* 4 year HPFS	43%
2-year OS	62%**	65%**	86%*	72%	62%	53%

*$p<0.05$, **Based on published Kaplan-Meier curves.

4-year survival (46% vs. 25%, $p = 0.04$) and hepatic disease-free survival (67% vs. 43%, $p = 0.03$) for the HAI FUDR and IV 5-FU arm compared with the resection alone arm.

- In a Memorial Sloan-Kettering Cancer Center (MSKCC) randomized study, 156 patients with resected hepatic metastases were randomized to systemic 5-FU/LV(Mayo schedule) or systemic 5-FU/LV(Mayo schedule) plus HAI FUDR and dexamethasone.[5] In contrast to the other randomized trials, patients in this study were only randomized after hepatic metastasis resection. Primary end points were 2-year progression-free and overall survival rates. Forty percent of patients had received prior adjuvant chemotherapy following resection of their primary CRC, and 15% had received prior chemotherapy for metastatic disease. Randomization was performed intraoperatively after complete resection of hepatic metastases, and patients were stratified based on number of metastatic lesions and prior treatment history. Ninety-two percent of patients received treatment as assigned. Two-year survival rate was 86% in the combined-therapy group compared with 72% for systemic therapy alone ($p = 0.03$), with median survivals of 72.2 and 59.3 months, respectively. Two-year hepatic progression-free survival rate was 90% for the combined and 60% for the monotherapy groups ($p < 0.001$). An updated hepatic progression-free survival rate at 5 years is 70% and 40% ($p = 0.0001$), respectively, and a median overall progression-free survival is 31 and 17 months ($p = 0.001$), respectively. Moderate toxicity was evidenced, with 39% of patients in the combined therapy group requiring hospitalization for diarrhea, neutropenia, mucositis or small bowel obstruction, compared with 22% of the monotherapy group ($p = 0.02$). Elevated bilirubin was seen in 18% of patients in the combined therapy arm. In most patients, the bilirubin returned to the normal range; however, 6% of patients required biliary stent placement. In the control group, 2% had an elevation in bilirubin and 2% required biliary stents. There was no significant difference between the arms in therapy-related deaths

(1 combined, 2 monotherapy). In an updated analysis, 57% of patients were alive in the combined group and 48% in the control group at 5 years and 41% and 27%, respectively, in the group receiving systemic therapy alone are alive at 10 years.[6]

- The previous two studies demonstrate lower hepatic and extrahepatic rates of recurrence for combined systemic 5-FU and HAI FUDR therapy after surgical resection (Table 6-2). The 2-year survival rate after liver resection (86%) was significantly better with the combined therapy in the MSKCC study, and compared favorably with adjuvant systemic therapy alone (72%) and with historical 2-year survival rates for patients treated with resection.[1,5,7–11]
- In contrast, a study by Lorenz et al. in the *Annals of Surgery* randomized 226 patients to surgery alone or surgery with HAI fluorouracil.[3] A scheduled interim analysis demonstrated no proven benefit to adjuvant HAI therapy in this trial, and therefore it was terminated early.
- Adjuvant HAI FUDR trials, combined with more active systemic chemotherapeutic and molecularly targeted agents including cetuximab and bevacizumab, are ongoing.

HAI Chemotherapy in Unresectable Liver-Only Metastatic CRC Patients

- Ten major prospective randomized clinical trials have been published comparing fluoropyrimidine-based HAI therapy to systemic chemotherapy in metastatic colorectal cancer patients with liver-only metastases (see Table 6-3).[12–21] Although most of these studies demonstrated a statistically significant superior response rate and improved disease-free survival with HAI chemotherapy compared to systemic chemotherapy alone, interpretation is difficult based on the availability of effective new agents such as bevacizumab and cetuximab.

Randomized Trials

- Two European trials conducted during the late 1980s randomly assigned patients to either best supportive care

Table 6-3: Randomized Trials of HAI Chemotherapy for Unresectable Liver Metastases

Study	Arms	n	n(%)receiving Assigned tx	Crossover to HAI	OR (CR+PR)	Median TTP(mo)	Median OS(mo)
MSKCC 1987	HAI FUDR	48	45 (94%)	Yes	50%*	9*	17
	IV FUDR	51	48 (94%)		20%	5	12
NCI 1987	HAI FUDR	32	21 (66%)	No	62%*	NR	17†
	IV FUDR	32	29 (92%)		17%	NR	12†
NCOG 1989	HAI FUDR	67	50 (75%)	Yes	42%*	NR	16.5
	IV FUDR	76	65 (86%)		10%	NR	15.8
City of Hope 1990	HAI FUDR	31	31 (100%)	Yes	55%*	8.8	13.8
	IV 5-FU	10	10 (100%)		20%	7.5	11.6
NCCTG 1990	HAI FUDR	39	33 (85%)	No	48%	6	12.6
	IV 5-FU/LV	35	36 (100%)		12%	5	10.5
French 1992	HAI FUDR	81	70 (87%)	No	44%*	NR	15*
	IV 5-FU or BSC	82	41 (50%) had 5-FU		9%	NR	11
English 1994	HAI FUDR	51	49 (96%)	No	NR	NR	13.5*
	IV 5-FU or BSC	49	10 (20%) had 5-FU		NR	NR	7.5
German 2000	HAI FUDR	54	37 (69%)	Yes	43%*	5.9	12.7
	HAI 5-FU/LV	57	40 (70%)		45%	9.2	18.7
	IV 5-FU/LV	57	52 (91%)		20%	6.6	17.6
MRC/EORTC 2003	HAI 5-FU/LV	145	95 (66%)	No	22%‡	7.7	14.7
	IV 5-FU/LV	145	126 (87%)		19%	6.7	14.8
CALGB 2003	HAI FUDR	68	59 (87%)	No	48%*	5.3	22.7*
	IV 5-FU/LV	67	58 (87%)		25%	6.8	19.8

*$p<0.05$, †based on published Kaplan-Meier curves, ‡responses were calculated at a single time point (12 weeks).

or HAI FUDR. French (Rougier et al.)[12] and English (Allen-Mersh et al.)[13] studies both demonstrated a survival advantage of HAI therapy, but most of the control patients did not receive systemic chemotherapy; hence, the survival advantage was predominately in comparison to best supportive care.

- The response rates of HAI-based therapy from these 10 randomized clinical trials ranged from 22–62%, compared with a range of 10–25% with systemic chemotherapy. Four of these 10 trials allowed for crossover to HAI-based therapy upon progression of disease, possibly masking any survival advantage of HAI-based therapy.[15–18] In addition, many patients did not actually receive HAI-based therapy even though they were included in the HAI subset using intention-to-treat analysis.
- The data of some of these trials have been subjected to two different meta-analyses.[22,23] Each meta-analysis confirmed the trends that were apparent in the individual studies—namely, that response rates were greater with HAI therapy.
- An English trial involving 290 metastatic colorectal cancer patients randomized to HAI 5-FU/LV or systemic deGramont schedule of 5-FU/LV demonstrated no statistically significant difference in response rates, progression-free survival, or overall survival.[14] Randomization was performed prior to hepatic arteriography, and 19% of the patients randomized to the HAI arm were precluded from HAI therapy secondary to abnormal hepatic vasculature. Overall, 37% of patients randomized to the HAI arm did not receive HAI therapy, compared with only 14% of the systemic chemotherapy patients. Among the patients who did receive HAI therapy, 29% of patients received fewer than six cycles due to catheter failure. These factors make interpretation of the trial difficult.
- A German cooperative group randomized oligometastatic colorectal cancer patients to three arms with HAI 5-FU/LV, HAI FUDR, or intravenous 5-FU/LV.[18] Despite the statistically significant doubling of the response rates of the HAI chemotherapy arms compared to the IV

5-FU/LV arm, this did not translate into a statistically significant survival advantage, perhaps reflecting the high (51%) crossover reported in the study. The reported systemic toxicity with 5-FU/LV was clearly greater than with FUDR, with much greater stomatitis and diarrhea in the 5-FU/LV arms.

- A Cancer and Leukemia Group B (CALGB) trial randomized metastatic colorectal cancer patients to either HAI FUDR, leucovorin, and dexamethasone or IV 5-FU/LV.[24,19] Patients found to have extrahepatic disease at exploratory laparotomy were treated with HAI therapy despite these findings to avoid selection bias, and crossover was not permitted for the 135 randomized patients. The primary endpoints of the CALGB trial were survival and a correlation with tumor biology. An assessment of clinical response and toxicity and an economic analysis were also performed.[19] Quality of life using the Rand 36-Item Health Status Profile, Memorial Symptom Assessment Scale, and other instruments demonstrated an improvement in physical functioning in the HAI group. A statistically significant survival advantage was seen in the HAI FUDR arm relative to the IV 5-FU/LV arm (22.7 vs. 19.7 months). The response rate was also much higher in the HAI arm at 48% vs. 25% ($p = 0.001$), as was the hepatic disease-free survival rate.

Conclusions

- Although there remains no debate that resection of oligometastatic disease leads to long-term survival and hence should be performed when possible, the optimal approach and regimen (neoadjuvant vs. adjuvant, regional approach plus systemic chemotherapy vs. chemotherapy alone, optimal chemotherapy regimen) remain unclear.
- With the success of new chemotherapeutic agents incorporating molecularly targeted agents, as demonstrated by the increasing published institutional series demonstrating significant anti-tumor responses leading to surgical candidacy of many patients who would previously have

been ineligible based on tumor distribution and burden, it is difficult to interpret older trials involving less effective chemotherapeutic regimens.

- For now, a multidisciplinary approach should be individualized for each oligometastatic CRC patient, with strong consideration of clinical trials involving systemic chemotherapy and/or a regional approach.

References

1. Fong Y, Fortner J, Sun RL, et al. Clinical score for predicting recurrence after hepatic resection for metastatic colorectal cancer: analysis of 1001 consecutive cases. *Ann Surg.* 1999; 230:309–18; discussion 318–321.
2. Schussler-Fiorenza CM, Mahvi DM, Niederhuber J, et al. Clinical risk score correlates with yield of PET scan in patients with colorectal hepatic metastases. *J Gastrointest Surg.* 2004;8:150–157; discussion 157–158.
3. Lorenz M, Muller HH, Schramm H, et al. Randomized trial of surgery versus surgery followed by adjuvant hepatic arterial infusion with 5-fluorouracil and folinic acid for liver metastases of colorectal cancer. German Cooperative on Liver Metastases (Arbeitsgruppe Lebermetastasen). *Ann Surg.* 1998;228:756–762.
4. Kemeny MM, Adak S, Gray B, et al. Combined-modality treatment for resectable metastatic colorectal carcinoma to the liver: surgical resection of hepatic metastases in combination with continuous infusion of chemotherapy—an intergroup study. *J Clin Oncol.* 2002;20:1499–1505.
5. Kemeny N, Huang Y, Cohen AM, et al. Hepatic arterial infusion of chemotherapy after resection of hepatic metastases from colorectal cancer. *N Engl J Med.* 1999;341: 2039–2048.
6. Kemeny N CA, Gonen L, Blumgart L, Fong Y. Updated Survival of Randomized Study of Hepatic Arterial Infusion(HAI) and Systemic Chemotherapy(SYS) Versus SYS Alone as Adjuvant Therapy after Resection of Hepatic Metastases from Colorectal Cancer, American Society of Clinical Oncology. Orlando, FL, 2005.
7. Nordlinger B, Guiguet M, Vaillant JC, et al. Surgical resection of colorectal carcinoma metastases to the liver. A prognostic scoring system to improve case selection, based on

1568 patients. Association Francaise de Chirurgie. *Cancer.* 1996;77:1254–1262.
8. Jamison RL, Donohue JH, Nagorney DM, et al. Hepatic resection for metastatic colorectal cancer results in cure for some patients. *Arch Surg.* 1997;132:505–510; discussion 511.
9. Scheele J, Stangl R, Altendorf-Hofmann A. Hepatic metastases from colorectal carcinoma: impact of surgical resection on the natural history. *Br J Surg.* 1990;77:1241–1246.
10. Fegiz G, Ramacciato G, Gennari L, et al. Hepatic resections for colorectal metastases: the Italian multicenter experience. *J Surg Oncol Suppl.* 1991;2:144–154.
11. van Ooijen B, Wiggers T, Meijer S, et al. Hepatic resections for colorectal metastases in The Netherlands. A multiinstitutional 10-year study. *Cancer.* 1992;70:28–34.
12. Rougier P, Laplanche A, Huguier M, et al. Hepatic arterial infusion of floxuridine in patients with liver metastases from colorectal carcinoma: long-term results of a prospective randomized trial. *J Clin Oncol.* 1992;10:1112–1118.
13. Allen-Mersh TG, Earlam S, Fordy C, et al. Quality of life and survival with continuous hepatic-artery floxuridine infusion for colorectal liver metastases. *Lancet.* 1994;344:1255–1260.
14. Kerr DJ, McArdle CS, Ledermann J, et al. Intrahepatic arterial versus intravenous fluorouracil and folinic acid for colorectal cancer liver metastases: a multicentre randomised trial. *Lancet.* 2003;361:368–373.
15. Kemeny N, Daly J, Reichman B, et al. Intrahepatic or systemic infusion of fluorodeoxyuridine in patients with liver metastases from colorectal carcinoma. A randomized trial. *Ann Intern Med.* 1987;107:459–465.
16. Hohn DC, Stagg RJ, Friedman MA, et al. A randomized trial of continuous intravenous versus hepatic intraarterial floxuridine in patients with colorectal cancer metastatic to the liver: the Northern California Oncology Group trial. *J Clin Oncol.* 1989;7:1646–1654.
17. Wagman LD, Kemeny MM, Leong L, et al. A prospective, randomized evaluation of the treatment of colorectal cancer metastatic to the liver. *J Clin Oncol.* 1990;8:1885–1893.
18. Lorenz M, Muller HH. Randomized, multicenter trial of fluorouracil plus leucovorin administered either via hepatic arterial or intravenous infusion versus fluorodeoxyuridine

administered via hepatic arterial infusion in patients with nonresectable liver metastases from colorectal carcinoma. *J Clin Oncol.* 2000;18:243–254.

19. Kemeny N ND, Hollis R. Hepatic arterial infusion (HAI) versus systemic therapy for hepatic metastases from colorectal cancer; a CALGB randomized trial of efficacy, quality of life (QOL), cost effectiveness, and molecular markers, ASCO, 2003;252.
20. Chang AE, Schneider PD, Sugarbaker PH, et al. A prospective randomized trial of regional versus systemic continuous 5-fluorodeoxyuridine chemotherapy in the treatment of colorectal liver metastases. *Ann Surg.* 1987;206:685–693.
21. Martin JK, Jr., O'Connell MJ, Wieand HS, et al. Intra-arterial floxuridine vs systemic fluorouracil for hepatic metastases from colorectal cancer. A randomized trial. *Arch Surg.* 1990;125:1022–1027.
22. Reappraisal of hepatic arterial infusion in the treatment of nonresectable liver metastases from colorectal cancer. Meta-Analysis Group in Cancer. *J Natl Cancer Inst.* 1996; 88:252–258.
23. Harmantas A, Rotstein LE, Langer B. Regional versus systemic chemotherapy in the treatment of colorectal carcinoma metastatic to the liver. Is there a survival difference? Meta-analysis of the published literature. *Cancer.* 1996;78: 1639–1645.
24. Kemeny N, Seiter K, Conti JA, et al. Hepatic arterial floxuridine and leucovorin for unresectable liver metastases from colorectal carcinoma. New dose schedules and survival update. *Cancer.* 1994;73:1134–1142.
25. Kemeny N, Conti JA, Cohen A, et al. Phase II study of hepatic arterial floxuridine, leucovorin, and dexamethasone for unresectable liver metastases from colorectal carcinoma. *J Clin Oncol.* 1994;12:2288–2295.

CHAPTER 7

Chemotherapy

Fluorouracil

- Fluorouracil (5-FU) has been the mainstay in the treatment of colorectal cancer since the 1950s, when it was first characterized by Dr. Heidelberg at the University of Wisconsin.
- Fluorouracil is an antimetabolite that works primarily by inhibiting the synthesis of thymine nucleotides by blocking the rate-limiting enzyme thymidylate synthase.
- It is generally combined with biomodulator leucovorin (folinic acid) to improve response rates; however, in a meta-analysis of nine trials comparing fluorouracil with or without leucovorin, the leucovorin-treated patients demonstrated no statistically significant overall survival advantage. Likely explanations for the lack of overall survival advantage include the small numbers of patients in these trials, the short duration of response in general to fluorouracil, and the high rate of crossover in these trials to the arms containing leucovorin.[1]
- Major side effects are directly related to the type of infusion schedule (bolus vs. protracted infusion), and include diarrhea, mucositis, cytopenias, and hand-foot syndrome (redness at palmar and plantar surfaces). See Table 7-1.
- Fluorouracil is administered in many different schedules; see Table 7-2.
- The Southwest Oncology Group (SWOG) "octopus" trial randomized patients to seven different treatment regimens with various doses of fluorouracil with and without leucovorin, and found no difference between any of the schedules.[2]
- Fluorouracil has a short half-life (< 10 minutes) and is S-phase dependent. Therefore, a protracted infusion, as

Table 7-1: Comparison of Toxicities from a Randomized Trial of Fluorouracil Schedules*

Toxicity	Bolus 5-FU	Continuous Infusion 5-FU
Mucositis	30.6	4.2
Diarrhea	23.5	3.2
Nausea	4.1	0.0
Alopecia	15.3	0.0
Plantar-palmar erythema	4.1	7.4
Neutropenia	53.1	1.1
Anemia	1.0	0.0
Infection	9.2	2.1

*Adapted from Ross PJ, and Cunningham D. Protracted infusion of 5-FU for colorectal cancer. *Management of Colorectal Cancer.* 1998, Martin Dunitz Ltd., London.

opposed to a bolus infusion, may affect more tumor cells as they progress through the cell cycle.

- The Meta-analysis Group in Cancer combined six randomized trials comparing continuous infusion fluorouracil to bolus fluorouracil. Both the response rate and the survival were improved with the continuous infusion schedule. The response rate increased from 14% to 22% and the survival increased from 11.3 months to 12.1 months ($p = 0.04$). Most importantly, the grade 3–4 toxicities were significantly higher in the bolus arms, particularly neutropenia (31% vs. 4%, $p < 0.0001$).
- A commonly used modern schedule for fluorouracil is an intermittent, high-dose infusion (DeGramont) schedule. This schedule infuses leucovorin first at 200 mg/m^2, followed by a bolus of fluorouracil at 400 mg/m^2, and then a 22-hour infusion of fluorouracil at 600 mg/m^2. The treat-

Table 7-2: Common Fluorouracil Schedules for Colorectal Cancer

Schedule	5-FU	Leucovorin
Weekly (Roswell Park schedule)	500 mg/m^2 IV weekly for 4 weeks on a 6 week cycle	500 mg/m^2 (high dose) or 20 mg/m^2 (low dose) IV weekly for 4 weeks on a 6 week cycle
Daily × 5 (Mayo Clinic)	425 mg/m^2 IV daily for 5 days on a 4 week schedule	20 mg/m^2 IV daily for 5 days on a 4 week schedule
LV5FU2	400 mg/m^2 IV bolus followed by a 22 hour infusion of 600 mg/m^2 on days 1 and 2 repeated every other week	200 mg/m^2 IV on days 1 and 2 repeated every other week

ment is repeated a second day, and then both days of chemotherapy are again delivered on a 2-week schedule. This schedule, known as LV5FU2, demonstrated a high response rate, a modest improvement in survival, and a favorable toxicity profile. More importantly, this schedule formed the basis for combination chemotherapy with oxaliplatin, a combination known as FOLFOX-4 (FOLinic acid, Fluorouracil, OXaliplatin 4). Subsequent modifications in the administration schedule of FOLFOX have been developed for convenience and possible enhanced responses. There are no prospective randomized trials comparing the major schedules of FOLFOX (4–7).

Capecitabine

- Capecitabine is an oral fluorouracil pro-drug, converted by the liver and tumor cells to the active 5-FU by a variety of enzymes, predominately by thymidine phosphorylase, which is present in high concentration in tumor cells, leading to the theoretical selective concentration of the active metabolite within tumor cells.[3]

- It is absorbed intact through the bowel mucosa.
- A practical benefit of an oral agent is the ability to mimic the pharmacokinetics of a protracted infusion schedule of chemotherapy without the need for permanent venous access and pump devices.
- Large clinical trials have demonstrated noninferiority of capecitabine to IV fluorouracil/leucovorin in the adjuvant and metastatic setting of colorectal cancer patients.[4,5]
- The toxicities of capecitabine are similar to prolonged-infusion fluorouracil, including mucositis, diarrhea, and hand-foot syndrome. Similarly, neutropenia is much less common than is seen with a bolus 5-FU schedule.

Irinotecan

- Irinotecan is a semisynthetic derivative of camptothecin, an alkaloid derived from either *Camptotheca acuminata* or *Nothepodytes foetida,* trees that are native to China. Irinotecan, through its active metabolite SN-38, works by inhibiting the nuclear enzyme topoisomerase I.
- A randomized trial comparing irinotecan to best supportive care reported by Cunningham et al. involving patients with prior fluorouracil therapy demonstrated nearly a 3-month statistically significant survival advantage of irinotecan compared to best supportive care.[6] Confirming this study is a trial by Rougier et al. in which the improvement in survival was more modest, at about 2 months.[7] These patients who had failed bolus fluorouracil, however, were randomized to irinotecan vs. continuous infusion fluorouracil.
- Two landmark studies confirm that irinotecan in addition to 5-fluorouracil/leucovorin is superior to 5-fluorouracil/leucovorin alone in the first-line treatment of metastatic colorectal cancer.[8,9] A randomized phase III trial by Saltz et al. compared bolus 5-fluorouracil and leucovorin with or without irinotecan. Clear superiority of irinotecan/5-FU/LV to 5-FU/LV alone was demonstrated with a near doubling of the response rate (28% to 50%) and improved median survival (12.6 months to 14.8 months, respectively). Another randomized crossover phase III trial by Douillard et al. also confirmed the superiority of an

Table 7-3: Common Schedules of Irinotecan, Fluorouracil, and Leucovorin

Schedule	Irinotecan	5-FU	Leucovorin
IFL	125 mg/m^2 IV over 90 minutes weekly for 4 weeks over a 6 week cycle	500 mg/m^2 IV weekly for 4 weeks over a 6 week cycle	20 mg/m^2 IV weekly for 4 weeks over a 6 week cycle
FOLFIRI	180 mg/m^2 IV over 2 hours every 14 days	400 mg/m^2 bolus followed by a 46-hour infusion of 2,400 to 3,000 mg/m^2 every 14 days	200 mg/m^2 IV over 2 hours every 14 days
Irinotecan single agent	350 mg/m^2 IV over 90 minutes once every 3 weeks		

irinotecan/5-FU/LV regimen to 5-FU/LV alone in response and survival utilizing an infusional 5-fluorouracil schedule. The addition of irinotecan improved median survival from 14.1 months to 17.4 months ($p = 0.031$).

- Major side effects of irinotecan include diarrhea, alopecia, cytopenias, nausea, and fatigue. The diarrhea has both an acute onset, managed with atropine during the infusion, and a delayed onset, typically managed with anti-diarrheal agents and antibiotics if necessary. Recommendations regarding the management of these side effects have been published from a panel formed to address toxicity concerns of these and other irinotecan trials.[10]
- See Table 7-3 for common administration schedules.

Oxaliplatin

- Oxaliplatin is a platinum compound that acts by forming adducts on DNA, interfering with replication and transcription.[11] It is more efficient at inhibiting DNA chain elongation, and forms adducts that are more hydrophobic than cisplatin or carboplatin. It may be these reasons why oxaliplatin appears to have a broad range of activity, greater than other platinum analogues, particularly in tumors that are resistant to cisplatin and carboplatin.

- Oxaliplatin has little activity as a single agent,[12–14] and is most commonly administered with 5-fluorouracil and leucovorin (LV5FU2) in a combination known as FOLFOX-4. The difference in response rate between oxaliplatin when administered as a single agent (approx. 10%) and with fluorouracil (46%–58%) is quite striking, suggesting a high degree of synergy between oxaliplatin and other chemotherapeutic agents.
- Large randomized studies have demonstrated an improved response rate with FOLFOX-4 compared to LV5FU2 alone.[15,16] In a pivotal study by de Gramont et al., 420 patients with untreated metastatic colorectal cancer were randomized to FOLFOX-4 or LV5FU2. The response rate of FOLFOX-4 was more than double that of LV5FU2 (51% vs. 22%, $p = 0.0001$); however, survival was not statistically different between the two arms, which may be related to second-line treatment. In the second study, by Giaccetti et al., the response increased from 16% to 53% ($p < 0.001$) with the addition of oxaliplatin. This study also failed to demonstrate a statistically significant improvement in overall survival with oxaliplatin. Because of this and other reasons, the approval of oxaliplatin in the United States was delayed until further studies confirmed the superiority of FOLFOX-4 over irinotecan with bolus 5-fluorouracil and leucovorin.
- A large, randomized multi-center trial compared three different regimens of oxaliplatin, irinotecan, and 5-fluorouracil in the first-line therapy of metastatic colorectal cancer patients. The initial design had only irinotecan treatments, and then the trial was amended to include the addition of oxaliplatin arms, and finally amended once again to exclude the treatment arms that had unfavorable toxicity profiles. The three remaining arms were oxaliplatin with infusional 5-fluorouracil and leucovorin (FOLFOX-4), irinotecan with bolus 5-fluorouracil and leucovorin (IFL), and irinotecan and oxaliplatin (IROX).

A total of 795 patients were randomized to the three therapies. All therapies had acceptable toxicities, but the FOLFOX-4 arm demonstrated superior response and survival compared to the IFL or IROX arms. The superior survival of the patients on the FOLFOX-4 arm must be tempered by the fact that oxaliplatin was not FDA-approved at the time of the trial, and hence, patients on the IFL arm infrequently received second-line oxaliplatin.[17]

- A prospective randomized clinical trial with crossover design comparing FOLFOX-6 and FOLFIRI, an infusional fluorouracil schedule with oxaliplatin or irinotecan, respectively, by Tournigand et al. demonstrated noninferiority of either regimen in the first-line setting. No differences in response rate, progression-free survival (PFS), and overall survival, as well as secondary PFS, were demonstrated.[18] The side effect profiles of the two were clearly different, suggesting that the choice of first-line regimen should be selected based on the tolerability of the underlying toxicity profiles.
- Oxaliplatin has also been combined with capecitabine, an oral analogue of 5-fluorouracil, in multiple different schedules.[19] Preliminary reports of a phase III trial of capecitabine and oxaliplatin compared to the infusional FOLFOX schedule have recently demonstrated tolerability and noninferiority in progression-free survival.
- Toxicities of oxaliplatin include peripheral sensory neuropathies (both acute and chronic), cytopenias, nausea, vomiting and allergic reactions with continued exposure.
- The peripheral neuropathies of oxaliplatin are both cold-induced acute neuropathies and persistent non-cold-induced. The infusion of calcium gluconate and magnesium sulfate (1 g) both prior to and after oxaliplatin has been shown to reduce grade 3 neuropathies (7% vs. 26%) with no effect on efficacy.[20] However, it remains unclear of its impact without large randomized trials.
- To date, many strategies have been investigated in an attempt to reduce the incidence of oxaliplatin-associated sensory neuropathy. This includes multiple neuromodulating agents including xaliproden, which have failed to

demonstrate an impact on the neurotoxicity in randomized phase III trials.
- See Table 7-4 for common schedules of oxaliplatin administration.

Cetuximab

- Cetuximab is a chimeric monoclonal antibody directed against the extracellular ligand-binding domain of the epidermal growth factor receptor, EGFr, overexpressed in over 70% of colon and rectal tumors.
- EGFr is a member of the erbB family of receptors, erbB1 (also known as EGFr), erbB2 (also known as Her2/neu), erbB3, and erbB4. These receptors form homo- and hetero-dimers, which subsequently activate the raf/mek/erk pathway, the AKT pathway, and other pathways leading to increased cellular proliferation and alterations in programmed cell death. Altering the signaling of EGFr has been shown to inhibit growth of colorectal cancer cell lines and is presumed to be an important pathway in tumorogenesis.
- In vitro, cetuximab has shown a high affinity to EGFr and has shown significant single agent activity. It has also been shown to be synergistic with a variety of other chemotherapy agents as well as with radiation.
- Preclinical data in irinotecan-refractory colon cancer xenograft models demonstrated evidence of anti-tumor activity with reversal of irinotecan resistance with the administration of both irinotecan and cetuximab. Based on this preclinical in-vitro and xenograft data and a single anecdotal report of a major response to cetuximab plus irinotecan in a young irinotecan-refractory patient, large multicenter randomized trials were performed to determine the clinical responses.
- In phase II trials in patients with irinotecan-refractory colorectal cancer, cetuximab has demonstrated a 10% response rate as a single agent and a 23% response rate when given concurrently with irinotecan (Saltz trials, BOND-1 Trial).[21,22] The median overall survival in these studies was not statistically significant between the arms

Table 7-4: Common Schedules of Oxaliplatin, Fluorouracil, and Leucovorin

Schedule	Oxaliplatin	5-FU	Leucovorin	Capecitabine
FOLFOX4	85 mg/m^2 IV over 2 hours on day 1 every other week	Similar to LV5FU2	Similar to LV5FU2	
FOLFOX6	100 mg/m^2 IV over 2 hours on day 1 every 14 days	400 mg/m^2 bolus followed by a 46-hour infusion of 2,400 to 3,000 mg/m^2 every 14 days	200 mg/m^2 IV over 2 hours every 14 days	
CapOx 7 day	85 mg/m^2 IV over 2 hours on day 1 every other week			3,500 $mg/m^2/d$ PO BID for 7 days every other week
CapOx 14 day	130 mg/m^2 IV over 2 hours on day 1 every three weeks			2,000 $mg/m^2/d$ PO BID for 14 days every three weeks

(8.6 months in the combination therapy vs. 6.9 months in the monotherapy group), although this likely reflects the fact that 50% of the patients in the monotherapy group received combination therapy with irinotecan upon progression.

- Currently, cetuximab is FDA approved only for colorectal cancer patients who have progressive disease after irinotecan administration.
- Side effects include infusion reactions and a generalized acneiform rash.
- Those with a more intense rash have been shown to be more likely to respond to therapy, with a response rate of 25.8% in those with a skin reaction vs. 6.3% for those without a skin reaction ($p = 0.005$).
- Hypomagnesemia has been demonstrated in patients receiving cetuximab, with the mechanism of action still under investigation, and hence magnesium levels should be routinely evaluated in patients receiving cetuximab.
- The use of cetuximab in the first-line setting in combination with FOLFOX and FOLFIRI and as adjuvant treatment with FOLFOX is currently being investigated by multiple clinical trials.
- Multiple institutional studies have demonstrated that cetuximab has objective clinical activity in EGFr-negative tumors.[23] Because the intensity of EGFr expression does not correlate with response to therapy, immunohistochemical EGFr testing is not warranted at this time. There are no surrogate markers for response to EGFr agents at this time.
- Cetuximab is administered weekly as an IV infusion. The loading dose is 400 mg/m^2, followed by 250 mg/m^2 thereafter. However, a recent pharmacokinetic study appears to support a biweekly schedule of 500mg/m^2, which is currently under evaluation in a prospective clinical trial.

Bevacizumab

- Bevacizumab is a recombinant, humanized monoclonal antibody directed against the VEGF ligand, with a half-life of approximately 21 days. The VEGF pathway plays a key role in tumor neovascularization.

- In colorectal cancer, an increase in angiogenesis has been associated with poor prognosis and increased risk of recurrent disease.[24]
- VEGF is thought to play an important role not only in tumor neovascularization, but also in the survival of existing immature VEGF-dependent tumor vasculature. A large prospective randomized trial demonstrated that bevacizumab added to IFL (bolus irinotecan, 5-fluorouracil, and leucovorin) improved response rates and survival compared with IFL alone.[25] In the trial, 402 patients were randomized to the arm containing IFL and bevacizumab, and 411 were randomized to receive only IFL. The IFL plus bevacizumab arm demonstrated superiority in both objective response (45% vs. 35%, $p = 0.004$) and overall survival (20.3 months vs. 15.6 months, $p < 0.001$) compared to the IFL alone arm. The only differential statistically significant toxicity in the bevacizumab arm was an increase in grade 3 hypertension, which was controlled with anti-hypertensive agents. A rare but serious toxicity included gastrointestinal perforations in six patients in the group receiving bevacizumab. These were thought to be related to either a response to treatment, recent bowel surgeries, or peptic ulcer disease. It is therefore recommended to use caution when administering bevacizumab near the time of surgery. Recent institutional matched-cohort studies appear to demonstrate that surgery can be performed safely 6 weeks after bevacizumab administration (two half-lives).
- Other rare but serious toxicities of bevacizumab include nephrotic range proteinuria and reversible posterior leukoencephalopathy syndrome (RPLS).
- A large randomized study by the Eastern Cooperative Oncology Group (ECOG 3200) demonstrated superior response and survival with bevacizumab plus FOLFOX-4 compared to FOLFOX-4 alone and to bevacizumab alone in the second-line setting of bevacizumab naïve, irinotecan, and 5-fluorouracil refractory colorectal cancer patients. A bevacizumab-alone arm reported a 3% response rate and, hence, single agent bevacizumab cannot be supported at this time.[26] Bevacizumab also received FDA approval in the second-line setting on the basis of this

trial. However, these patients were bevacizumab naïve in the second-line setting.

- The role of continued bevacizumab administration after failure of a first-line bevacizumab-containing regimen remains unclear, with several trials currently addressing this clinical question.
- Bevacizumab is commonly administered bi-weekly as an IV infusion at 5 mg/kg.

Panitumumab (Vectibix)

- Panitumumab is a humanized monoclonal antibody against EGFr, recently FDA approved in the salvage setting, based on an international randomized phase III trial comparing single agent panitumumab to best supportive care. This trial, involving 463 patients receiving panitumumab every 2 weeks, demonstrated a 46% decrease in tumor progression rate versus best supportive care alone ($p < 0.000000001$).
- The current clinical role of panitumumab in practice remains unclear. Large randomized trials in the first- and second-line setting of metastatic colorectal cancer will be reported in the near future to further define its clinical utility.

Combinations of Biologic Therapy

- The BOND-2 trial addressed the feasibility and, in a preliminary manner, efficacy of bevacizumab added to cetuximab alone or cetuximab plus irinotecan in patients with irinotecan refractory disease.[27] Preliminary data were encouraging, with a 23% and 38% RR and a 6.9 and 8.5 month Time to Tumor Progression (TTP),[27] respectively, which appear significantly better than historical controls from the BOND-1 trial (11% and 23% RR, 1.5 and 4 months TTP).[22,27] It should be noted, however, that this is a small trial with 39 and 35 patients, respectively, reported in each arm in this preliminary report. Ninety percent of the patients in this study also previously received oxaliplatin, making the combination an effective salvage regimen. No unexpected grade 3/4 toxicities were discovered.[27]

First-Line Chemotherapy

- Currently, there are many choices for first-line therapy including infusional fluorouracil with irinotecan or oxaliplatin and capecitabine/oxaliplatin regimens. Fluoropyrimidine regimens (5-fluorouracil and capecitabine) in combination with oxaliplatin or irinotecan with bevacizumab or cetuximab have been explored in phase II trials and recently reported in phase III trials. A recently reported large prospective randomized 2 × 2 phase III first-line colorectal trial comparing FOLFOX to XELOX (capecitabine/oxaliplatin) with second randomization involving placebo or bevacizumab has demonstrated noninferiority of XELOX relative to FOLFOX, and statistical PFS advantage to the addition of bevacizumab. This 2,000-patient clinical trial with a median follow-up of 18.6 months reported a progression-free survival (PFS) of 8 months with XELOX and 8.5 months with FOLFOX. Furthermore, the addition of bevacizumab to chemotherapy improved PFS compared to chemotherapy alone (9.4 months vs. 8 months, $p = 0.0023$).
- Hence, first-line treatment should be determined individually for each patient, based on the toxicity profiles and individual patient needs. Please see Table 7-5 for a list of median overall survival for various first-line therapies.
- Grothey et al. analyzed data from multiple randomized phase III studies to determine the importance of the availability of all three chemotherapeutic agents in the treatment of metastatic colorectal cancer.[28] In this report, patients who received combination therapy up front had an improvement in survival by 3.5 months. Further, as the percentage of patients who received all three chemotherapies (fluorouracil-leucovorin, irinotecan, and oxaliplatin) increased, the overall survival increased, a statistically significant correlation at $p = 0.008$.
- Multiple randomized phase III clinical trials are currently enrolling metastatic colorectal cancer patients to further

Table 7-5: Median Overall Survival for First-line Colorectal Cancer Therapies

Regimen	Survival (months)
MFOLFOX6, then FOLFIRI	20–21
FOLFIRI, then FOLFOX6	20–21
IFL and bevacizumab	20–21
FOLFIRI	17
FOLFOX4	16
IFL	14–15
Infusional 5-FU/LV	14–15
Capecitabine	12–13
Bolus 5-FU/LV	12–13
No therapy	4–6

advance the standards of care. Examples include the Intergroup trial (FOLFIRI or FOLFOX chosen by treating investigators' discretion with randomization to one of three arms: cetuximab, bevacizumab, or both agents), the U.S. Oncology Trial (FOLFOX/bevacizumab vs. infusional 5-FU/LV/cetuximab/bevacizumab), and the Crystal (cetuximab) and PACCE (panitumumab) trials.

Second-Line and Third-Line Therapies

- With two highly active regimens containing irinotecan or oxaliplatin, the best second-line therapy should include a non-cross-resistant regimen not utilized in the first-line setting. FOLFIRI has a fairly low response rate as a second-line agent, however, at only 4%.[18] This low response rate, however, did not influence the survival of patients who received this treatment as second-line therapy.

- Cetuximab is FDA approved for colorectal cancer patients who have failed irinotecan therapy, and hence is currently a good choice for third-line treatment in combination with irinotecan.
- Unfortunately, salvage data presented at the American Society of Clinical Oncology meeting in 2004 demonstrated that 5-FU/LV/bevacizumab in bevacizumab-naïve patients failing prior oxaliplatin and irinotecan has a dismal 1% response rate.[29]
- Panitumumab was recently FDA approved for use in colorectal cancer patients in the salvage setting failing prior 5-FU/LV, oxaliplatin, and irinotecan.
- Phase I-II trials, as available, should be strongly considered for patients with good performance status who have failed standard chemotherapeutic agents including 5-FU/LV, oxaliplatin, irinotecan, and cetuximab.

Novel Agents in Colorectal Cancer

- Novel agents currently being explored in this disease include the VEGF pathway modulator PTK787 and the fully humanized EGFr antibody panitumumab. These explore targets already known to be effective in colorectal cancer. Other agents, including the kinesin spindle protein inhibitor SB715992, microtubule inhibitor epothilone D, IGF receptor antagonists, TRAIL inhibitors, her1/2 inhibitors, and multiple other pathways, are being pursued in the treatment of colorectal cancer.

References

1. Advanced Colorectal Cancer Meta-Analysis Project. Modulation of fluorouracil by leucovorin in patients with advanced colorectal cancer: evidence in terms of response rate. *J Clin Oncol.* 1992;10:896–903.
2. Leichman CG, Fleming TR, Muggia FM, et al. Phase II study of fluorouracil and its modulation in advanced colorectal cancer: a Southwest Oncology Group study. *J Clin Oncol.* 1995;13:1303–1311.
3. Schuller J, Cassidy J, Reigner BG, et al. Tumor selectivity of Xeloda in colorectal cancer patients. *Cancer Chemother Pharmacol.* 2000;45:291–297.

4. Van Cutsem E, Twelves C, Cassidy J, et al. Oral capecitabine compared with intravenous fluorouracil plus leucovorin in patients with metastatic colorectal cancer: results of a large phase III study. *J Clin Oncol.* 2001;19:4097–4106.
5. Hoff PM, Ansari R, Batist G, et al. Comparison of oral capecitabine versus intravenous fluorouracil plus leucovorin as first-line treatment in 605 patients with metastatic colorectal cancer: results of a randomized phase III study. *J Clin Oncol.* 2001;19:2282–2292.
6. Cunningham D, Pyrhonen S, James R, et al. Randomised trial of irinotecan plus supportive care versus supportive care alone after fluorouracil failure for patients with metastatic colorectal cancer. *Lancet.* 1998;352:1413–1418.
7. Rougier P, Van Cutsem E, Bajetta E, et al. Randomised trial of irinotecan versus fluorouracil by continuous infusion after fluorouracil failure in patients with metastatic colorectal cancer. *Lancet.* 1998;352:1407–1412.
8. Douillard JY, Cunningham D, Roth AD, et al. Irinotecan combined with fluorouracil compared with fluorouracil alone as first-line treatment for metastatic colorectal cancer: a multicentre randomized trial. *Lancet.* 2000;355:1041–1047.
9. Saltz L, Cox J, Blanke C, et al. Irinotecan plus fluorouracil and leucovorin for metastatic colorectal cancer. *N Eng J Med.* 2000;343:905–914.
10. Rothenberg ML, Meropol NJ, Poplin EA, Van Cutsem E, Wadler S. Mortality associated with irinotecan plus bolus fluorouracil/leucovorin: summary findings of an independent panel. *J Clin Oncol.* 2001; 19:3801–3807.
11. Fichtinger-Schepman AM, Baan RA, Luiten-Schuite A, et al. Immunochemical quantitation of adducts induced in DNA by cis-diamminedichloroplatinum (II) and analysis of adduct-related DNA unwinding. *Chem Biol Interact.* 1985; 55:275–288.
12. Machover D, Dias-Rubio E, de Gramont A, et al. Two consecutive phase II studies of oxaliplatin (L-OHP) for treatment of patients with advanced colorectal carcinoma who were resistant to previous treatment with fluoropyrimidines. *Ann Oncol.* 1996;7(1):95–98.
13. Levi F, Perpoint B, Garufi C, et al. Oxaliplatin activity against metastatic colorectal cancer. A phase II study of 5-day continuous venous infusion at circadian rhythm modulated rate. *Euro J Cancer.* 1993;29A:1280–1284.

14. Rothenberg ML, Oza AM, Bigelow RH, et al. Superiority of oxaliplatin and fluorouracil-leucovorin compared with either therapy alone in patients with progressive colorectal cancer after irinotecan and fluorouracil-leucovorin: interim results of a phase III trial. *J Clin Oncol.* 2003;21:2059–2069.
15. De Gramont A, Figer A, Seymour M, et al. Leucovorin and fluorouracil with or without oxaliplatin as first-line treatment in advanced colorectal cancer. *J Clin Oncol.* 2000;18:2938–2947.
16. Giacchetti S, Perpoint B, Zidani R, et al. Phase III multicenter randomized trial of oxaliplatin added to chronomodulated fluorouracil-leucovorin as first-line treatment of metastatic colorectal cancer. *J Clin Oncol.* 2000;18:136–147.
17. Goldberg RM, Sargent DJ, Morton RF, et al. A randomized controlled trial of fluorouracil plus leucovorin, irinotecan, and oxaliplatin combinations in patients with previously untreated metastatic colorectal cancer. *J Clin Oncol.* 2004;22:23–30.
18. Tournigand C, Andre T, Achille E, et al. FOLFIRI followed by FOLFOX6 or the reverse sequence in advanced colorectal cancer: A randomized GERCOR study. *J Clin Oncol.* 2004;22:229–237.
19. Scheithauer W, Kornek GV, Raderer M, et al. Randomized multicenter phase II trial of two different schedules of capecitabine plus oxaliplatin as first-line treatment in advanced colorectal cancer. *J Clin Oncol.* 2003;21(7):1307–1312.
20. Gamelin L, Boisdron-Celle M, Delva R, et al. Prevention of oxaliplatin-related neurotoxicity by calcium and magnesium infusions: a retrospective study of 161 patients receiving oxaliplatin combined with 5-fluorouracil and leucovorin for advanced colorectal cancer. *Clin Cancer Res.* 2004;10:4055–4061.
21. Saltz L, Hochster H, Rubin M, et al. Cetuximab (IMC-C225) plus irinotecan (CPT-11) is active in CPT-11-refractory colorectal cancer (CRC) that expresses epidermal growth factor receptor (EGFR). *Proc Am Soc Clin Oncol.* 2001;20:3a.
22. Cunningham D, Humblet Y, Siena S, et al. Cetuximab monotherapy and cetuximab plus irinotecan in irinotecan-refractory metastatic colorectal cancer. *N Engl J Med.* 2004;351:337–345.
23. Chung KY, Shia J, Kemeny NE, et al. Cetuximab shows activity in colorectal cancer patients with tumors that do not express the epidermal growth factor receptor by immunohistochemistry. *J Clin Oncol.* 2005; 23:1803–1810.

24. Reinmuth N, Parikh AA, Ahmad SA, et al. Biology of angiogenesis in tumors of the gastrointestinal tract. *Microsc Res Tech.* 2003;60:199–207.
25. Hurwitz H, Fehrenbacher L, Novotny W, et al. Bevacizumab plus irinotecan, fluorouracil, and leucovorin for metastatic colorectal cancer. *N Engl J Med.* 2004;350:2335–2342.
26. Giantonio BJ, Catalano PJ, Meropol NJ, et al. High-dose bevacizumab in combination with FOLFOX4 improves survival in patients with previously treated advanced colorectal cancer: Results from the Eastern Cooperative Oncology Group (ECOG) study E3200. Abstract #169a presented at the ASCO Gastrointestinal Cancers Symposium, June 2005.
27. Saltz LB, Lenz H, Kindler H, et al. Interim report of randomized phase II trial of cetuximab/bevacizumab/irinotecan (CBI) versus cetuximab/bevacizumab (CB) in irinotecan-refractory colorectal cancer. 2005 Gastrointestinal Cancers Symposium Abstract #169b.
28. Grothey A, Sargent D, Goldberg R, et al. Survival of patients with advanced colorectal cancer improves with the availability of fluorouracil-leucovorin, irinotecan, and oxaliplatin in the course of treatment. *J Clin Oncol.* 2004;22:1209–1214.
29. Chen HX, Mooney M, Boron M, et al. Bevacizumab (BV) plus 5-FU/leucovorin (FU/LV) for advanced colorectal cancer (CRC) that progressed after standard chemotherapies: an NCI Treatment Referral Center trial (TRC-0301). *Proc Am Soc Clin Oncol.* 2004;23:249.

CHAPTER 8

Management Issues Specific to Rectal Cancer

Surgery

- Surgery is an essential part of therapy for patients with localized rectal cancer.
- Total mesorectal excision (TME) has been shown to improve local recurrence rates and should be considered standard practice in multiple clinical trials, most of them retrospective.[1,2] One such study compared TME with conventional surgery at different hospitals in the United States, Norway, the United Kingdom, Japan, and the Netherlands. A total of 1,411 patients were analyzed. Patients either received a TME (in the United States and United Kingdom), a D3 lymphadenectomy (in Japan), or conventional surgery (Norway and the Netherlands). Despite the many limitations in this cross-institutional comparison, there was a 30% survival difference and 25% local recurrence difference favoring those who had the TME and D3 lymphadenectomy. Current rectal cancer trials now require a TME as standard therapy.

Chemotherapy

- Therapy for rectal cancer around the time of surgery includes either preoperative chemotherapy and radiation (neoadjuvant) or postoperative chemotherapy and radiation (adjuvant). Survival rates of the two modalities are the same; however, a randomized trial comparing preoperative therapy vs. postoperative therapy showed improved tolerability and local control rates with neoadjuvant treatment.[3] In this large, randomized study, over 800 patients were randomized to either preoperative chemotherapy (120-hour continuous intravenous infusion at a dose of 1,000 mg/m^2 per day during the first and fifth weeks of radiotherapy) with 50.4 Gy radiation or the same chemotherapy and radiation delivered after surgery. Both groups received four 5-day cycles of adjuvant fluorouracil after the planned surgery or chemoradiation. The overall survival of the two groups was similar, 76% and 74% for the preoperative and postoperative treatments, respectively. The local control rates were different, however, with a 6% local recurrence rate in the preoperative group and 13% in the postoperative group ($p = 0.006$). This may have been due to the inability to administer the planned therapy in the postoperative group due to excess toxicities. Only 54% of the postoperative patients received the complete course of radiation therapy. This compares to 92% of the preoperative patients receiving the complete course of radiation therapy. Certainly the grade 3 and 4 toxicities seen postoperatively were significantly higher, at 27% vs. 40% for preoperative patients.

- Preoperative therapy should be administered to all patients with stage II and III rectal adenocarcinomas, T3 or greater tumors, or node-positive tumors. This is in contrast with colorectal cancers, where stage II tumors do not routinely receive adjuvant therapy.
- Fluorouracil remains the standard of care, given concurrently with radiation. Ongoing studies are evaluating the use of irinotecan, oxaliplatin, and biologics; however, these have not yet shown improvement over fluorouracil as a single agent in phase III studies.
- Further cycles of adjuvant fluorouracil chemotherapy are also recommended after surgery and radiation, usually to complete a total of 6 months of therapy.
- Continuous infusion fluorouracil has been shown to be better tolerated than bolus fluorouracil. In a randomized study published in the *New England Journal of Medicine* in 1994, the treatment arm with a continuous infusion of fluorouracil not only was better tolerated, but also resulted in a significantly greater overall survival and relapse-free survival than the arm with the bolus 5-FU. The recommended dose for continuous infusion 5-FU is 225 $mg/m^2/day$ IV during the entire course of radiation.[4]

Radiation

- Standard dose radiation consists of 5,040 cGy delivered in fractions of 180 cGy per day, 5 days per week.
- For those with metastatic disease, local radiation can control rectal pain and bleeding. Pain is decreased in 80% of those treated, and bleeding can be controlled in approximately 70% of those treated.
- Radiation should also be considered for patients who have local recurrence, if radiation was not part of the original treatment.

References

1. Kapiteijn E, Marijnen CAM, Nagtegaal ID, et al. Preoperative radiotherapy combined with total mesorectal excision for resectable rectal cancer. *N Engl J Med.* 2001;345:638–646.
2. Havenga K, Enker WE, Norstein J, et al. Improved survival and local control after total mesorectal excision or D3 lymphadenectomy in the treatment of primary rectal cancer: an international analysis of 1411 patients. *Eur J Surg Oncol.* 1999;25(4):368–374.
3. Sauer R, Becker H, Hohenberger W, et al. Preoperative versus postoperative chemoradiotherapy for rectal cancer. *N Engl J Med.* 2004;351:1731–1740.
4. O'Connell MJ, Martenson JA, Wieand HS, et al. Improving adjuvant therapy for rectal cancer by combining protracted-infusion fluorouracil with radiation therapy after curative surgery. *N Engl J Med.* 1994;331:502–507.

Index

F

G

H

I